Eczema and Allergy -

THE HIDDEN CAUSE?

My Story by
JENNIFER WORTH SRN,SCM

Second edition

Special Contributors:
Professor Anthony Frew BChir,MB,MA,MD,FRCP
Dr John Mansfield MRCS,LRCP,DRCOG
Dr Helen McEwen MBBS,MRCGP

Publishing history

Eczema and Food Allergy - the Hidden Cause?
was first published in 1997 by Merton Books
ISBN 1 872560 02 4
Copyright © Jennifer Worth 1997

A revised and updated edition was produced by Merton
Books in 2003 for sale on-line at www.allerbuys.com
Copyright © Jennifer Worth 2003

Second edition revised and updated, published by
Merton Books 2007 and reprinted 2012

Copyright © Jennifer Worth 2007

ISBN 978-1-872560-18-2

MERTON BOOKS
PO Box 279
Twickenham TW1 4XQ
020 8892 4949
www.mertonbooks.co.uk

Acknowledgements

I would like to extend my grateful thanks to:
my dear husband, Philip
Pat Schooling, editor of Merton Books
Patrick Mackarness
Drs Michael Radcliffe, Len McEwen, Helen McEwen
Sybil Birtwistle and Michael Price
Pearl Skofield, healer, St John's Church Healing Group, Boxmoor
Alison Whyte, Features Editor, *Nursing Times*
Suzannah Hart
and to all the many other people who have expressed interest and
offered help and advice.

Publisher's Note

This book describes dietary programmes which are sometimes severely restricted. It would be most inadvisable for any reader to attempt an elimination diet without appropriate medical supervision. The author's own diet was closely supervised by her medical adviser and she strongly urges others to seek similar professional help.

This book is *not* intended for the treatment of children, who are still growing and for whom an elimination diet would be inappropriate.

Contents

PART I

MY STORY

It happened over a
period of time. This is
how Jennifer's suffering
began and grew to
encompass her whole
body. It nearly drove her
to suicide.

Chapter 1

MY STORY

This book is intended as a message of hope to all those suffering from severe eczema.

My family is riddled with asthma. About 50% of all members of the family suffer from asthma, and I have had it since childhood. Asthma has been identified by the medical profession as an allergic condition but no-one has ever suggested to me, or to any member of my family, to my knowledge, that the cause or the allergy should be sought and treated. My asthma was always treated with drugs.

Over a period of time, in 1990 and 1991, the eczema started. Like "the cloud no bigger than a man's hand" which eventually covered the sky, two little itchy spots appeared on my legs, and wouldn't go away. I had no idea what they were, and assumed they were insect bites. But no, they were the ominous beginnings of a hideous skin disease, eventually covering my entire body, which nearly drove me to suicide. I think that if I had not met the doctor who eventually cured me, I would have committed suicide. Unlike most people, I have never had the slightest fear of death. I fear suffering, I fear helpless old-age and I certainly fear being unable to die, but death itself I have always regarded as the best and truest friend that we have. The old expression goes "while there is life, there is hope". But on a deeper level, I say "while there is death, there is hope".

But I digress. Two tiny itching spots on my legs – that was all to begin with. But they got larger and itchier, and similar spots appeared on my arms and shoulders, telling me that they were not insect bites. I saw an acupuncture doctor who recognised the spots for what they were, eczema, and told me that he could cure it. He tried for six months to do so, but with no success. The eczema just spread slowly, insidiously, over my arms and legs.

Eventually, he told me that I needed cortisone treatment, and my GP arranged for me to go to the skin clinic at our local hospital. The consultant dermatologist confirmed that I had atopic eczema, and told me it was incurable, and the only treatment available was cortisone creams and ointments. I was reluctant to start steroids, but the consultant told me that my skin was far worse than that of the average person who came to their clinic (in fact at that time it was only a tiny part of what it later became!) and that steroids were the only treatment. I agreed to start, thinking in my naivete that it would be for a limited period, and that I would be weaned off them later. This was not to be the case.

I mentioned the word "allergies" to the doctor. She told me that it was most unlikely that I was allergic to anything at all, but agreed that a patch test should be done on my skin, just to see. The test proved negative to everything, and the consultant's opinion was vindicated. I was dubious about this, because I have always been highly allergic to cats.

The original diagnosis "atopic eczema" is interesting. What is the meaning of "atopic"? It took me a long time to find out. Literally it comes from the Greek, meaning "of no fixed place". It also means, medically, an inborn disposition, or tendency to develop allergies. This tendency is inherited, running in families. Not all members of the family are afflicted and, in some people, the allergic reaction may start in babyhood, or it may start for the first time in adult life. The cause (the allergen) and the effect (the reaction) can and will vary widely in different members of the same family (hence the Greek "of no fixed place"). An unpleasant allergic reaction to all sorts of everyday things is very common. In some people, however, who are highly atopic, allergies to many things can develop causing severe illness.

I said that the diagnosis of "atopic eczema" is interesting. The expression is used so often that one hardly hears or reads the word "eczema" without the word "atopic" attached to it. Then why, if eczema is known to be of atopic origin, is it not automatically treated as an allergic reaction to something and the allergen sought out and eliminated? Why should a highly trained consultant dermatologist tell me in one breath that I have atopic eczema and in the next breath that it is highly unlikely that I am allergic to anything at all?

The consultant dermatologist at the hospital persuaded me to use a strong steroid cream twice daily. Within a short time, the eczema appeared to have cleared up. I would say "appeared" because anyone looking at me would say my skin was quite clear, but I knew it was not. I could feel it under the skin, somehow bubbling up and being pushed back all the time by the cream. If at any time I omitted to cover a small area of skin with the cream, that area would erupt within a few hours. However, to all appearances my skin was clear and after about four months of out-patient visits, the doctor discharged me. The cortisone cream was to be continued at the same strength twice daily; there was no suggestion of weaning me off it, as I had anticipated. In fact as I put my hand on the door to leave, the consultant spoke the ominous words: "You will probably be on cortisone now for the rest of your life".

These words had a profound affect on my thoughts, and on my subsequent life. It was a cold February day, and I had about a mile to walk home, but that mile in a cold drizzle was very important to me. I reflected all the way home on those words. I knew very little about eczema at that time, but I had heard that in many instances the use of steroids proves to be a downward spiral of stronger and stronger creams for less and less benefit. I knew that steroid creams, although applied to the skin, are absorbed into the blood stream. As a nurse and medical Ward Sister of eighteen years' experience, I had seen cases of steroid overdose and the devastating effects this can have on the body. I knew perfectly well that steroids taken in any way will adversely affect the natural immune system of the body.

Before reaching home, I had come to my decision. I would not be on cortisone creams for the rest of my life.

Having been on cortisone creams for four to five months I decided to wean myself off over a period of three months. I was still on a strong cream. I first cut down the amount on each application for about two to three weeks, then asked my own GP to prescribe a weaker steroid, which I used twice daily for another two to three weeks. Then I reduced the quantity of each application. Finally, I cut down to once a day application. The eczema was certainly coming back and quickly. Patches on my arms and legs were showing signs of a red rash, which was very itchy.

Then a most significant thing happened, about eight to ten weeks after starting reduction of the steroids. I caught a very severe stomach bug and I did not eat for four days. The eczema cleared completely, and I used no steroids at all.

I had never heard of food allergies, in spite of 18 years working in hospitals. In fact if I had been told, I would probably not have believed the information, as many people do not believe it today. But the eczema had quite gone during the four days without food. However, a stomach bug passes fairly quickly and you are hungry when you feel well again. As soon as I started eating again the eczema returned, in exactly the same places as before. It was very near the end of my planned three month withdrawal of steroids, so I decided to withdraw them completely at that time. The month was April, and I had been discharged from the hospital in early February.

I told my doctor about the experience of the stomach bug and she said it was probably coincidence, that natural remissions are known to occur in eczema, which could easily account for it vanishing for a few days. I did not think it was coincidence or natural remission. I thought it was highly significant, and that the eczema must be related to food. I determined to start looking into my diet.

At the time I had very little knowledge of eczema, no knowledge at all about diet or food allergies, and I didn't know where to start. I had joined the National Eczema Society, and so wrote to them asking for any information they could send me about food allergy causing eczema. The reply stated that there is little or no connection between eczema and food. An article by an eminent dermatologist which was enclosed with the letter said the same thing, and stated that some children are allergic to certain foods, but not adults. I just did not believe it. My own experience told me otherwise. However, the article said that children can be allergic to milk – so I decided to take milk out of my diet. It made no difference at all.

I started hunting for books on allergies, particularly food allergies. I found quite a number in the library, and in the local health food shop, but depressingly none of them contained more than a few paragraphs about eczema and food allergy and several of these books said there was no connection, as the article had stated.

I tried experimenting by myself. I put myself on what would normally be called "a healthy diet", high in fresh foods, whole grains, brans, brown rice, fruit and vegetables, yogurt. I cut out tea, coffee, alcohol and most foods with additives in them.

In retrospect the first mentioned foods were all the wrong things for me. "A healthy diet" is not the same thing as looking for things to which you are allergic. But I did not know this at the time. The only sensible thing I achieved was to cut out all stimulant drinks and especially food additives.

There are now something over 4000 chemical food additives used in our food production. That is in addition to fertilisers, pesticides, fungicides, insecticides and all the bombardment of chemicals that are sprayed on to all growing crops, both before and after harvesting. Other than organic food, there is almost nothing that can be bought which is free from adulteration of some sort or another. No wonder the incidence of food allergies is increasing. No wonder allergic diseases are increasing both in incidence and in severity.

The diet achieved no improvement in my skin. It didn't get worse, but it did not improve either. There remained an itchy red rash on my legs and arms.

In early June (about six weeks after withdrawing the steroids completely) I embarked on a course of reflexology treatment. My reason for doing so was logical – I had rejected the medical treatment of steroids and so when a reflexologist told me that her treatment could help, if not cure the eczema, I did not hesitate to go for it.

It did not help. In fact my skin became rapidly worse, spreading within a few days from my arms and legs to my entire body. The speed with which this developed was quite frightening. I submitted to four treatments, encouraged to do so by the assurance that the eczema has got to get worse before it gets better and that it would go away after the fourth treatment. After each weekly treatment, I felt and looked worse. First one leg and then the other began to swell, from the thigh to the feet. My skin turned a deep purple/reddish colour and began sloughing off. The glands in my groin came up like a bunch of hard purple grapes.

Pints of water collected in my legs. I have always had the legs of a ballet dancer, but now they looked like elephant's legs – huge and completely solid from thighs to ankles. I lay with my legs higher than my head all night to try to drain them. This was successful and in the mornings my legs were back to their normal shape. To achieve this transformation during the night and early morning I had passed huge quantities of urine. Many times (almost with detached interest) I weighed myself before retiring and then again in the morning. There was a swing of between 10-14 lbs in my body weight, before and after the fluid had drained away.

The next two to three months were a nightmare. I felt and looked terrible. My concentration level was so low that sometimes I could scarcely conduct a rational conversation. I felt so weak and ill and shaky, I could scarcely creep about. And the itching….

The itching, day and night, like a million tiny insects crawling around under the skin, biting and nibbling beneath the skin surface. It is impossible to imagine the horror of it, if you have not experienced it. It is absolutely impossible to stop yourself from scratching, frantic, hysterical scratching that goes on and on for hours. The itch seems deep in the tissues, and you scratch harder and harder in order to get at it, until you have drawn blood. Then it begins to hurt, but the pain is infinitely preferable to the itching.

Many nights I spent the entire night crying and scratching. Usually I fell asleep from exhaustion around dawn, to wake up a few hours later with the sheets sticking to my body. Then they had to be pulled off, or washed off, which would start the cycle of itching again.

I know a woman whose mother, with severe eczema, clawed a great piece of flesh out of her throat; the scar was still visible 30 years later. I saw a picture of a little girl of three who had scratched away half her cheek – the blood was running down her neck. I met a man who looked as though he had tried to pull his ears off his head. Perhaps he had, poor soul. They did not look like ears, grotesque red-brown lumps of raw flesh and scabs.

Nothing can stop the scratching and there is nothing that you can put on the skin or take internally to stop the itch. The skin becomes deformed and ugly. It thickens and mine quickly came to look and feel like thick red bubble plastic. The amount of fluid oozing out was quite astonishing. Many times, in the space of a few hours, I used up entirely a new kitchen roll, just mopping up the water that was seeping out of my body. The wet stage and the dry stage would follow each other on different parts of my body. When an area dried up, the skin would start to flake off, continuously for days on end. I quite calmly thought I would die. I thought to myself, "if you pull the bark off a tree, it will die. If all my skin comes off, I will die also". I was not the slightest bit afraid or regretful.

The work of washing and vacuuming seemed endless and I felt so weak. All my clothes and bed linen had to be washed every day, sometimes several times a day. I have never done so much washing in my life, even when I had two babies! I continuously needed to be vacuuming to get up the flakes of skin that were shedding off my body all the time.

I felt and looked disgusting and the smell was horrible. My husband was an angel. I could not have managed without him. He would hold me gently in his arms, and stroke my hair to comfort me. One day I was standing before my mirror crying, because I realised that my hair was coming out and my eyebrows also. He came into the bedroom unexpectedly, and took me in his arms. I burbled something about: "I can't bear looking such a mess". He said: "My darling, you are as beautiful to me today as you were the day we married". I cried all the more, this time from gratitude and love.

The only thing I found that could alleviate the itching was ice or very cold water. Frequently, I would put my arms into the freezer and rub them round the edges of the box. It calmed the worst itch for a time. But I could not put my whole body into the freezer, so I formed the habit of filling the bath with cold water before I went to bed, so that it was ready to plunge into when a frenzy of scratching threatened to get quite out of control. Water from the cold tap at three in the morning can be very cold in summer and near to freezing point in the middle of winter. But it did not feel cold, it felt glorious and I rejoiced as the cold, cold water spread over my back, shoulders and chest, where I had been driven mad with itching a few moments before. I relaxed and began to feel calm and drowsy. If there had been heavy snow, I swear I would have gone outside in the middle of the night to lie naked in the snow. Perhaps it is as well that there was no heavy snow, because I have heard that death from exposure is not at all unpleasant; you do not feel cold but the opposite, warm, content and drowsy, just as I felt, up to my neck in cold water in the middle of the night in the middle of January.

Nights were always worse. If I did go to sleep early in the night, I would wake myself up scratching – even through bandages, and with cotton gloves on. I had other nocturnal habits. I would prowl around the house doing odd jobs such as the ironing or cleaning the larder or sewing – anything to keep my hands busy so that I could not scratch myself. No-one knew how much of each night I was active, because of course I could not sleep with my poor husband.

I had another nocturnal habit – food bingeing. Apparently (I only learned this subsequently) a craving for the foods that you are allergic to is absolutely symptomatic of food allergies. It is called hidden or masked food allergy. The body seems to desire most that which is going to harm it most, and this strange phenomenon is noted over and over again by specialists in food allergies. My particular craving in the small hours of the morning was for hot porridge with cream and honey. I would make myself a huge bowl of it and eat the lot with relish. I felt better for it, the itching subsided and I felt content and comfortable. I really felt it did me good. I would go back to bed and sleep – but only for a few hours. I would usually wake up with a terrible jerk in a frenzy of scratching that could only end in drawing blood.

But enough of these grizzly details. This is a story of triumph, a message of hope. In spite of all the suffering, I did not for one moment doubt that somehow, some way I would find a complete cure. I just did not believe the prognosis that eczema is incurable. Nor did I resort at all to cortisone, because I knew that my condition was so bad that I would have to take it internally, as well as a very strong cream all over my body, which I knew would make things worse in the long run. I was taking a risk, because if infection had entered the skin, I would probably have developed blood poisoning, which very likely would have killed me. But I kept myself very clean, and generalised infection did not hit me.

One Sunday morning, in church, our lady priest was preaching. She was talking about the woman who had been bleeding for fourteen years, who touched the hem of Christ's robe in order to be healed, and was healed in that instant. She said: "Our Lord Jesus Christ still heals today, in just the same way, sometimes immediately, sometimes slowly, but prayers are never left unanswered".

In that moment, I knew that I must find a spiritual healer and through the Association of Spiritual Healers, I was able to contact a lady who lives near me, and who came to see me. As soon as she entered the door, I felt the presence of someone quite exceptional. Calm, goodness, purity, strength – all these things seemed to radiate from her, and she hadn't said a word!

We talked about my illness and the background to it.

Then she prayed for me, laying hands on all parts of my body and praying meanwhile. It took about an hour to do this. Afterwards, I slept for hours, not itching at all, which in itself is healing. She came to me once a week, every week for about a year, spending about an hour in prayer. The effect was always the same. In all the weeks and months that followed, I became absolutely dependent on her. She and my dear husband were the two people who kept me going. I may say that after the first session, I said to her "How much do I owe you?" (I was thinking of the average "alternative therapist" fees). She said: "Oh my dear, nothing at all, of course not, you can pay my petrol money, if you like!"

I had not witnessed, let alone experienced, spiritual healing before, and knew nothing about it. I can only say that somehow, there is a force of energy that can be channelled by a gifted healer, and conveyed to someone in need. I do not know what it is, but it is there, and it is powerfully effective.

I was not healed instantly, but slowly month by month, a slight improvement showed. However, a change in my attitude occurred almost instantly. I somehow felt that all the suffering I was going through was for a purpose. I did not know what, I could not see ahead, nor could I see a way to cure myself, but I knew somehow that I had to go through the suffering for a purpose to be achieved. This had a powerful effect upon everything. I no longer raged and cried aloud to the empty night - why, why, why me? A still small voice had whispered: "Be still and know that I am God, that I am with you even unto the ends of the earth". I have always been a deeply religious Christian, with a close affinity to professed sisters, or nuns. I have always known that acceptance of the will of God, as it is apparent in life, is a cornerstone of faith. I have always known that suffering is one of the great creative forces in life. I have always known these thing intellectually. Now I had to know them in actual daily living.

Not for one second did I accept that this hideous eczema would be with me for the rest of my life. That is not Christian acceptance. That is some sort of fatalism or defeatism. No, I simply knew that I would find a cure, but that I had to go through the worst of the disease for an undefined purpose to be fulfilled. I knew also that a hand would guide me every step of the way.

I continued searching for a cure in alternative medicine. I first saw a homeopathy doctor. He was obviously concerned about my condition, and said that he could not treat the skin until I was somewhat better in my general health. He gave me twenty-one powders of Morgan-Bach flower remedies, to take one potion per day for twenty-one days. He cautioned me particularly about cleanliness and avoiding infection – but I knew that anyway. He gave me some advice about food, (I had told him about my stomach-bug incident). Some of the advice was good – to avoid foods containing salicylates, about which he gave me a lot of useful information. I think that the Morgan-Bach powders did me some good, because I certainly felt stronger after twenty-one days. After that, he prescribed some tablets for my skin. They may have done me some good in the early stages, but after a change of prescription, the new tablets definitely made me worse, and I was itching and scratching madly after each dose, so much so that the skin of my legs completely broke down again. I took homeopathic medicines for about six months with no improvement.

I saw an aromatherapist, which made the skin worse, much worse, causing stinging and burning as well at itching. I did not know, and neither did the aromatherapist, that essential oils, which are powerful, can be harmful to the skin.

"It's some impurity in your heart coming out of your body through the skin," cried another therapist in triumph. "Perhaps it's some deep resentment or bitterness towards someone in the past that has been festering inside you, and is coming out now." I said I held no resentment towards anyone. "Ah, but you must, dear, it's so deep you are not aware of it, but it's an impurity that has got to come out." I was furious, but then she played into my hands – good. "What makes you angry, dear?" she whispered sweetly. I had to pause to control my rage. "Ignorant quacks like you, who play with the suffering of others, make me angry," I said, and left.

I tried hypnotherapy. Perhaps I am not a very good subject for hypnotism, because I just couldn't take the man seriously. In fact I giggled as I was coming round from his hypnotism which rather spoiled things, because he was obviously taking himself very seriously indeed.

I saw a Chinese herbal doctor. She would not give me any internal drugs to take as at the time I was taking homeopathic medicines. She prescribed some cream for me, but it had no effect whatever.

I tried urine therapy, a couple of drops placed under the tongue to be absorbed sub-lingually. The theory is that if you have a disease, antibodies will develop to fight it. Some of these antibodies will be passed in the urine, and if they are reintroduced into the bloodstream, by sub-lingual absorption, they will boost the immune system. There is no synthetic equivalent. Urine therapy is widely practiced in the orient, particularly for wound healing by direct application and is reputed to be effective, especially for burns.

The effect for me at first was excellent. Several open weeping sores on my arms healed over and the itching stopped. But the benefit wore off, and the nightmare started all over again. Nonetheless I think urine therapy should be researched more.

I tried the old-fashioned coal-tar bandages. They had a wonderful effect on my legs, so the nurse at our health centre applied them all over my body. I was trussed up like a mummy for two days and nights. The effect was miraculous. When the bandages came off, the swelling of my legs was gone and the eczema had completely cleared from my chest and stomach. However, so capricious is eczema, that when I tried the same treatment a few months later, it made the skin worse, not better!

The summer was glorious. Hot sun for weeks on end. Thank God I did not have to work full time. I still felt as weak as a kitten; I still itched all over and spent most of every night awake; my concentration level was very low still and I found it difficult to communicate with others. But at least I did not have the pressure of full time work. I had a loving husband and no anxieties, and a lovely garden to lie in, and every week the healer came to see me, giving me the strength to go on.

In November 1994, after three years from the onset of the disease, my anguished prayers were answered. I met Dr Tony Matthews, who was a retired pathologist and a member of the British Society for Ecological Medicine.* He had had allergies himself; had studied allergy-related diseases all his professional life, and had successfully treated patients with eczema.

I told him about my experience with a stomach bug and not eating for four days. He took me seriously. He was the first doctor to do so. He said: "Put yourself in my hands, and once we have found the right diet, the eczema will begin to clear within three to four weeks. I have never had a failure."

At that time known as the British Society for Allergy, Environmental and Nutritional Medicine.

⌘

Chapter 2

LEARNING ABOUT ALLERGIES

I had been fiddling around with diet ever since the stomach bug episode, but with no success at all. I have since met others with eczema who have done the same and the total lack of success leads them to conclude that food plays no part, or at best a very small part, in the cause and cure of eczema. This is the current opinion of the National Eczema Society, so the doctors and dermatologists of that society must have had the same experience with their patients.

This is not the case at all. Eczema is of atopic origin. That means that it is of allergic origin. There are only four sources of allergic reactions:

INHALED – airborne things

CONTACT – things touching the skin

INGESTED – food, drink, drugs

INJECTED – insect stings, things penetrating the skin, drugs.

Any one of these can cause eczema or dermatitis in varying degrees of severity, and with some people (not all) ingested allergens are going to cause the most trouble.

This has proved to be the case with me, and I cannot believe that I am unique. Quite a few doctors that I have spoken to have told me that my experience is very rare indeed. But I do not believe this.

Dr Tony Matthews arranged for a RAST (radioallergosorbent) test to be taken on me. This is a blood test which ascertains the presence or otherwise of IgE (Immunoglobulin E) in the blood when certain foods are taken. It is only partly reliable (sometimes it can give a false negative). It is only available on medical orders.

Tony told me that I must eat fresh cooked foods only, and eliminate from my diet the following:

- ☐ All processed, tinned, packaged, pre-cooked, dried, frozen foods

- ☐ All tea, coffee, alcohol, fruit juices – any bottled drink

- ☐ All tap water

- ☐ All medicines and drugs (I wasn't having any, anyway)

- ☐ All milk and milk products (including margarine)

- ☐ Eggs

- ☐ Cereal grains – wheat, corn, maize, rye, oats, barley, millet, brans

- ☐ Beef, veal and chicken

- ☐ Fish, shell fish, crustacea

- ☐ Soya and all legumes, pulses, beans, lentils etc.

- ☐ Fruit, especially dried fruits

- ☐ Vegetables containing pips or seeds

- ☐ Potatoes and tomatoes

- ☐ Spicy, hot, strong tasting or herb ingredients, including pepper

- ☐ Yeast, yeast extract (Marmite etc.) mushrooms, vinegar

- ☐ Sugar and all sweet things, including honey

- ☐ Nuts and seeds

- ☐ Chocolate including chocolate drinks.

He told me it was necessary to eliminate so much because of the likelihood of my being multi-allergic. He told me to cook everything.

My first reaction was: "My God, what am I going to eat? There's nothing left." The answer was tersely: "Yes there is. You can eat most meats and most vegetables and rice, you can eat as much as you like – don't let yourself go hungry. This will be a perfectly adequate diet and will keep you going for years. Anyway, it may not be necessary for long. Once your skin begins to clear you can start reintroducing."

All my life I have been a vegetarian and I told him this. He simply said: "Well, you have got to eat meat; you will need the protein." He said nothing more on the subject, and neither did I, but I privately decided that I would not eat meat, and that I could live quite well on vegetables alone.

Tony went on to explain many important things to me. At the time, they seemed a bit far-fetched, and implausible, but as the weeks and months passed and as I grew more accustomed to this strange new life style, the wisdom of these remarks rang true for me. He told me that if I am allergic to something then a very small amount of that food will affect me just as badly as a large amount.

He told me to be careful of sublingual absorption. Apparently tiny particles of anything can be quickly absorbed into the blood stream from under the tongue, in fact quicker than if it is absorbed from the stomach and the intestines. "For this reason," he said, "don't suck anything or chew anything, like chewing gum; don't lick stamps or envelopes, don't suck your pen when you are writing."

He told me to clean my teeth only with bottled water, and not to use standard toothpastes. When I asked why, he said: "Because for one thing you will absorb sublingually molecules of tap-water, which might be harmful. Secondly, most commercial toothpastes are made up from a cornflower paste and many other ingredients which you will absorb sublingually – like peppermint or colourings and preservatives. Use salt, or just bicarbonate of soda. Throw away your old toothbrush, because it will be contaminated, and buy a new one."

I asked Tony if I could have goat's-milk instead of cow's milk. He advised against it, because apparently, there is a cross-reaction from cow's milk, to both goat and sheep's milks. If you are allergic to milk, this will include all animal milks. He also said, in this connection, that the reason for not eating beef or veal is because in this country we commonly drink cow's milk and there is usually a cross-reaction between the milk and the animal from which it comes. I refrained from saying that I wouldn't be eating beef or veal anyway, so it did not apply.

He went on to say that many people are allergic to eggs, particularly egg white and if one is eliminating eggs, one must also eliminate chicken, because there is a cross-reaction between the eggs we commonly eat and the bird that lays them. I wasn't particularly interested in milk or eggs, and I had no interest at all in beef or chicken, but I was desperately interested in fruit. All my life I have loved fruit of every sort, and I have eaten loads of it. I was desolate at the idea of giving up fruit, even for a short time. I felt I couldn't live without it. I was prepared to argue the case. How could fruit be bad for anyone? Fresh fruit is so healthy, so good for you – everyone says so.

He patiently explained that, although this is an area that has not been properly researched, it seems that it is the pippy plant foods that cause most of the trouble for people with eczema. All fruit contains pips. I protested: "But you don't eat the pips, you throw them away." "Nevertheless," he said, "the fruits containing the pips are definitely allergenic and this has been shown time and time again. Also all grains, seeds and nuts come into the same category."

This group of foods is the widest single group of foods, and the group that I was most reluctant to eliminate.

It contains:

- ☐ All grains
- ☐ All fruits
- ☐ Some vegetables (cucumber, marrow, peppers etc.)
- ☐ All nuts
- ☐ All seeds such as caraway, sesame, sunflower etc.
- ☐ All dried fruits
- ☐ Peas, beans, lentils, pulses, soya beans
- ☐ Coffee, chocolate and carob (which are all derived from beans)

All my favourite things! If I had not been desperate, I would not have given them up, even for a short time.

I asked Tony about yeast. He explained that yeast is well known to cause a wide range of allergenic illnesses. "But why mushrooms and vinegar?" I said. "What's the connection?" "Well, yeast is a natural fungus and so are mushrooms. Spores from all the moulds or fungi will aggravate eczema. If you eat this fungus, it will have the same effect. Vinegar is included because it is a hidden source of yeast. Alcohol contains yeast, and vinegar is made from sour alcohol."

The thought of giving up honey was almost as bad as giving up fruit. I ate little sugar, but I love honey. Why honey? Everyone says it is good for you, and one therapist whom I had consulted about my eczema advised me to take a lot of Royal Jelly which is a special, expensive sort of honey, which she said would cure my eczema.

Tony said that this was quite wrong, and he explained to me the candida connection. I had never heard of it before. He said we all have in our intestines millions of microflora, which are beneficial to the body, and also fungal parasites, called candida albicans, which are kept in check, or in balance, by the microflora. In many people the microflora have become weak and ineffective, allowing the fungal parasites to breed in numbers. They then penetrate the gut wall and enter the bloodstream, at the same time allowing all sorts of molecules from undigested food to enter the blood stream causing multiple health problems.

I asked him how this could happen. "Well no-one really knows, but the overuse of antibiotics and the over-consumption of sugars has a lot to do with it, in my opinion." He looked at me severely. "The fungal spores feed on sugar and carbohydrates – which is one of the reasons why you must eliminate them. And that reminds me – don't take any medicines if you get a cold or flu, they all contain sugars. They all contain aspirin too, which is an irritant to eczema. And don't take antibiotics."

Tony was very strict about not drinking tap water, which is full of chemicals. These are harmless for most people, but can be dangerous to some people who cannot tolerate chemicals.

Tony told me I must clean up my house. I felt somewhat offended by this. "Well I do my best, and it seems pretty clean to me." He glared at me, "That's just the trouble. It's too clean. Chemically clean. We are filling our homes with chemicals and then wonder why we get ill. You will have to purge your house of all chemical washing powders, soaps, perfumes, sprays etc. There is no point in conducting an elimination diet if you are surrounded by toxic chemicals."

He gave me an excellent booklet produced by the British Asthma Campaign*, about chemicals in the home, and advised me to contact The Healthy House* about obtaining substitutes. He also advised me to join Action Against Allergy*, who can offer good advice on this subject, and all aspects of allergic disease. He said rather dryly: "You had better learn as much as you can about allergic diseases, because you will have to help yourself. You will get precious little help from my profession – medicine – though I am sorry to say it."
*See Useful Addresses section.

My first consultation with Tony ended with some very good advice: "An elimination diet can make you feel ill at first in unexpected ways, such as headache, dizziness, depression. These are withdrawal symptoms. Take no notice. It will pass."

We arranged to meet in a fortnight and I was left to get on with my diet.

I was in trouble right from the beginning because of my vegetarianism, which dates from earliest childhood. I have memories of sitting in a high chair, kicking and screaming and spitting out the meat that adults were trying to insist that I should eat. At school I remember sliding bits of meat off my plate into my lap when no-one was looking and hiding them up my knicker leg, to be disposed of in the playground – little girls wore bloomers with elasticated legs in those days. I cannot remember any adult who understood or sympathised with my aversion. I was just regarded as being awkward. When I was old enough to leave home I resolved to eat no more meat.

The habit and conviction of a lifetime cannot be reversed overnight. I was nauseated at the idea of eating animal flesh, and resolved just to eat vegetables. However, with no milk, cheese, eggs or fish; no beans or lentils, soya or nuts, no bread or grains, problems quickly developed – I was having no protein.

Within a few days, I had constant diarrhoea. Half an hour or less after eating a meal, I evacuated whatever I had eaten. I wouldn't have thought it possible to evacuate undigested cabbage or carrot within half an hour of eating them, but that is what I was doing. In two weeks I lost two stone of weight. I looked seriously ill and felt very weak.

I did not see Tony for a fortnight after starting the diet and when he saw me he was shocked and obviously very worried. I told him what I had been doing. He did not actually call me a fool, but the way he looked left no doubt as to what he was thinking. He simply said, "You have got to eat meat, or give up the attempt to cure your eczema this way. You have no alternative."

So I started eating meat for the first time in my life and from that moment things began to improve. The diarrhoea stopped, I gained a little weight and I felt stronger. Now I know that I need meat just as one knows that one is thirsty and needs a drink. But I never take it for granted. Every meal I say grace and a special benediction for the animal that has been killed for me to eat and be cured.

Then the first of many accidents happened. Trying to eliminate allergenic foods is full of pit-falls, which you cannot foresee. Tony had told me that elimination has got to be total. There can be no compromise at all, a tiny particle of a substance to which you are allergic can cause a reaction. Such reactions are more marked after a period of abstinence. He had told me this earlier but I didn't realise quite how absolute and unbending the elimination had to be.

I cooked roast duck for family dinner one Sunday three to four weeks after starting the diet. I stuffed the duck with a bread and onion stuffing. I had not eaten any bread for about a month, and I did not eat any stuffing. During the night I was driven frantic with itching and scratching. The next day my face was hideous and my body suppurating all over. I was in despair. I did not know what had caused it. I saw Tony and we went through the foods I had eaten during the 24 hours previously and he told me that the trouble must have been caused by the stuffing. I protested that I had not eaten any, but he told me that the molecules of the wheat would have permeated the duck and would have caused the flare-up. It took about a week for that flare-up to subside, and since then I have been rigorous in the detail of cooking and what has to be avoided.

After the roast duck incident, and the appalling reaction, I was more scrupulous about contamination of my meat and vegetable diet, which is based on what is called the Stone Age Diet or the hunter/gatherers diet.

This has an interesting theory behind it. It was first introduced by a Dr Richard Mackarness.* He found that most of the patients he saw were allergic to corn/wheat grain products or to milk and milk products or both. From this observation, he developed the theory that both of these foods are a relatively recent introduction to man's diet. When I first heard this I laughed and protested that mankind has been eating wheat for thousands of years. Ah, yes! But that is relatively recent in man's history, which goes back at least two or three million years. Prehistoric man was a hunter. He killed the animals that he ate. He was also a gatherer – he collected wild plant foods, which he ate. He was not a sower and reaper.

It takes a very long time for mutation to change an animal and a few thousand years is not sufficient time for everyone to be able to tolerate the new grain foods. Some people may still become allergic to them. The same is true of milk. Prehistoric man did not drink the milk of wild animals. It was only with the domestication of animals (about the same time as grain farming began) that it was possible. Not everyone can tolerate milk because they have not had enough time to adapt to it. Today the majority of the black race peoples cannot tolerate milk.

I thought this was all very far fetched when I first heard it, but the more I think about it the more sense it makes. Meat was the staple diet of homo sapiens when he came down from the trees and started to live in hunting communities and it must therefore be the food to which we are best adapted.

This, however, does not account for the "gatherers" stage of man's development. If man has been gathering nuts and fruits for two or three million years, why has he not adapted? Why are nuts and seeds potent allergens, and most fruits a source of trouble for eczema sufferers? Again there is a theory which explains this. All plants

---

*The late Dr Mackarness was a psychiatrist practising at Basingstoke General Hospital in the 1950s when he identified the link between food and health and its role in allergies. He promoted the Stone Age diet in his book *Eat Fat and Grow Slim*. His subsequent book *Not All in the Mind* (now out of print) is regarded as a classic. He left the NHS and pioneered Britain's first obesity and allergy clinic in the 1970s.

have chemical protective agents in them: eg. the fumes of onion, the sting of stinging nettles, the poison of laburnum. Atopic people are definitely allergic to all sorts of plants. This is readily observable: pollens cause hay fever, many plants cause rashes on the skin and watery eyes etc. These are contact and inhaled allergies, and are not far away from the assertion that many plant foods, when eaten, can and do cause allergic illnesses in many highly atopic people.

As mentioned earlier, I am a communicant Christian. One Sunday, just as I was taking the communion wafer at the altar, I realised that it was made from wheat! I asked Tony about this – could it harm me? "Of course it can," he said. "A weekly dose of wheat could keep your eczema bubbling along very nicely."

Shortly before Christmas I decided to go to the hairdresser to make myself look a bit better, for everyone's sake. "If my hair looks nice," I thought, "perhaps it won't matter that my face is red." It was disaster. God knows what they spray onto women's hair these days! It started off badly because my skin felt prickly after a few minutes in the salon. Whilst under the dryer I thought I would go mad with itching – but you can hardly tear your clothes off and scratch yourself all over in a chintzy little ladies' hair salon! Nor can you tear yourself free and rush out into the street when your hair is wet and all trussed up in curlers! I just had to stick it out. The hairdresser was obviously shocked when she turned off the dryer, and when I saw myself I was horrified. My poor face was not just red, it was deep crimson, and all swollen around the nose and the eyes, which were watering. However, it did not take long for it to subside. A good walk in the fresh air and the swelling and excessive redness had gone. This proves to me that contact allergens are less damaging to my skin than ingested allergens, because if I eat something and have a bad flare-up it will take about three days to subside.

Christmas came, and I hope I was not too much of a drag on everyone. I did not feel well, my skin was no better (even though it was about four to five weeks after starting the diet) and I was on a diet that made Christmas cooking difficult to say the least. Inevitably when you are surrounded by a lot of people merry-making mistakes are going to occur. I remember I ate a tiny bit of marzipan, a couple of dates, a spoonful of cranberry sauce with the turkey, at different times during the Festival. My skin flared up like a volcano – I wouldn't have thought it possible but it did. Unhappy, sleepless nights left me exhausted and tetchy. "Thank God I am the grandmother and not the mother of these little angels who never give you a moment's peace," I thought to myself.

It was shortly after Christmas that I was talking to Tony about my lack of sleep. He asked if I take anything at night and I told him that I took 25mg Phenergan because it makes me drowsy and as it is an antihistamine I hoped it would reduce the itching, although it didn't seem to. He said, "That may be, in part, the cause of the trouble; Phenergan might be made up in a cornflour base. There is no point in eliminating cereal grains from your diet, if you are taking corn every night in tablet form." He enquired from the manufacturers and sure enough Phenergan is produced in a corn base, which holds the tablet together. Phenergan linctus is produced in a sugar base, so that was out also.

He advised me to take calcium at night. Apparently calcium is a natural sedative, which used to be given as a sleeping tablet to patients in hospital wards. (Nursing textbooks of around 1910 advise the sedative effects of calcium, but today the benefits have been forgotten as many new drugs have been developed). Tony said "Take one at night, and you will begin to feel all woosey, and drop off to sleep." I took his advice and from that moment my sleeping improved. However, Tony warned that calcium must be taken with magnesium in a ratio of 2 parts calcium to 1 part magnesium. If calcium is taken alone it will disturb the biochemical balance of the body, and prevent the absorption of magnesium, which is essential to muscular function.

January was a miserable month. The weather was foul, and my skin was deteriorating again. Weeping eczema was again developing on my arms and legs, and the itch was intensifying. Particularly distressing were patches appearing on my face again which had been clean for months. My scalp was again affected, and hair started to fall out for the second time.

Eczema started to develop in my nose and ears, which had not happened before. This is particularly horrid because your nose feels as though it is running all the time, and so you wipe it, and that makes it worse, and you have to wipe it again, and yet again. Painful crusts develop up each nostril, which protrude, looking unsightly not to say disgusting; or which bleed and you are not aware of it, until you realise that someone is looking at you in horror and disgust.

The ears become engorged and inflamed and deep red, which itch like mad. You try to pull them off your head to stop the itch. I developed a severe ear infection from continually poking and scratching my ears. Again thoughts of death haunted me. To sleep, to die, to be free of torment. Heaven must be a place where there is no eczema.

I continued a strict diet. It is amazing that I did not just abandon the whole thing. I saw Tony again. He did not speak for a long time, but just looked at me steadily, then said: "What are you eating now?"

"Nothing but what you told me to eat:

☐ Meat

☐ Cooked green vegetables (but no pippy things)

☐ Cooked root vegetables (but not potatoes)

☐ Rice

☐ A little olive oil

☐ Sea salt

☐ Natural spring water."

"And what else? Little tastes of this or that, eh?"

"Nothing." (I was beginning to get cross.) "I have followed your instructions to the letter. I never cheat. I never make a mistake. There is no contamination because I cook for myself, and am scrupulously careful."

"What about other allergens, inhaled or contact?"

"I have anti-allergenic bedding, a centralised vacuum system, a water softener, electric cooking and central heating, no carpets in the bedroom, all cleaning materials are anti-allergenic, I wear only cotton or silk next to the skin. Above all I am on this foul diet which is doing no good."

Tony said nothing at all. He looked at my arms and legs, my entire body. He humphed and muttered to himself. Then he said: "I think you are allergic to the entire plant family. You must eat an all meat diet for a while."

I gasped in dismay. "Oh no, please. I couldn't."

"You must, if you are to cure the eczema."

"But why? I have eaten plant foods all my life."

"That's just the trouble. Allergies develop to commonly eaten foods. It is most unlikely that you are allergic to meat, because you have never eaten it. Also, the candida connection comes into it. Let me see your tongue."

I stuck my tongue out.

"As I thought, it is white. This indicates a fungal overgrowth throughout your entire alimentary system, which will enter your blood stream. The fungal parasites feed on fermenting plant foods and carbohydrates. They cannot feed on meat, because it does not ferment. You must eat meat only for a while."

With a heavy heart I returned home and discussed it with my dear husband, who said: "Try it, you have nothing to lose."

28

Reluctantly I cut out everything but meat and water. Within three days there was a marked improvement. Within three weeks my skin was clear.

The eczema had gone. After three years of suffering, of near insanity from perpetual itching, of near suicide from despair – the eczema had gone. I was delirious with joy. No words can describe the ecstasy in my heart – only a fellow eczema sufferer could understand. I behaved like a child, running around singing and laughing all the time and inviting people to look at me. They must have thought I was mad! I was – mad with relief and thankfulness.

Of course my poor skin was covered in scar tissue, which took weeks to heal. The hard lumps under the skin took several months to go completely. I was quite red, compared to most people. But my face rapidly cleared, and the crusts up my nose went. The eczema was not erupting from under the skin surface. Above all the intense itching had gone. Each day was very heaven to be alive and not to itch.

Tony was nearly as happy and excited as I was and we celebrated with a glass of Vichy water. He told me that he wanted me to see Professor Jonathan Brostoff in London, and that he would make an appointment. He told me to continue a meat only diet, but he was concerned about my weight, which had gone down another stone. I looked all skin and bones.

"How much fat do you eat?"

I said that I ate none, because I did not like it, it made me feel sick.

"You have got to eat fat," he said sternly. "Fatty acids are essential to the body. You cannot survive without them."

He then told me that meat fat, which has an undeserved bad reputation these days, is necessary for human tissue, particularly the brain cells and the motor neurone cells. The human race developed on eating animal flesh, and you can be quite sure that our hunter ancestors did not cut off and throw away all the fat, as we do today.

Tony told me to eat one third of fat to two thirds of lean meat at each meal. He said: "You will never be hungry if you eat like this. Your weight will remain low, but stable, you will never put on excess weight. You will have an increase of vitality and energy also. It is not animal fat that makes people over-weight and sluggish, it is an excess of refined carbohydrates and sugars that do the damage." He gave me a remarkable book to read, Eat Fat and Grow Slim by Richard Mackarness. I quote from page 50:

The Calorie Fallacy

There is a case for saying that a change from a vegetarian, gatherer's diet to one of animal meat and fat determined the change from apehood to manhood.

During the two to three million years that man has walked upright, he has been a hunter for nine-tenths of that time, subsisting on infrequent, large meals of animal tissue. Only in the last 6000 years has he eaten a high cereal diet and only in the last 100 years a diet high in refined starch and sugar and increasingly contaminated with chemical additives – substances made in the laboratory and never presented to the body chemistry before. Is it surprising that our bodies and brains, evolved as they were on natural fat and protein, are now showing adaptive breakdown in the face of new foods with which they are not equipped to deal?

Man comes at the end of mammalian evolution. His nearest rivals are all dying out and he has been left on top thanks to his highly developed and specialised nervous system. The brain and the nerves are made very largely of structural fats, unsaturated fats called phospholipids, and of proteins, few of them able to be synthesised from simpler chemicals in the body. All these essential fats and proteins must be provided ready-made in the diet. So man has evolved as a predator.

Looking at the earliest predators, some of the single-celled organisms which ate other single cells to acquire complex molecules which they could not make for themselves, we can see the advantages of such a way of eating. It makes room on the cellular genetic tapes for further specialisation if you cut out the instructions for making a complex vitamin like B12 by eating the B12 in a simpler cell which has made it for you.

So too with man the predatory meat-eater. Instead of getting the unsaturated fats and proteins essential for the building of his brain by laboriously collecting seeds, insects and green shoots, he eats the flesh of a herbivore which has already made these essential substances from plant food, and in one mouthful gets more brain-food than he would in a day's gathering in the forest.

This is how the idea of 'essential' foods came in. Whilst algae can make all their own nutrients from the simple salts and other chemicals dissolved in the water in which they float, more than 40% of the components of our cell membranes and nervous system must come from food – and the best and most concentrated source is other animals, fishes and birds.

So man must have essential fats and proteins, with other essential amino-acids, in his diet if he is to grow a good nervous system and arterial tree, and keep them in good shape into old age. The importance of dietary fat, especially the unsaturated fats which contain essential fatty acids which the body cannot make for itself, is now generally recognised. It is now known that these essential fatty acids are important for the formation of the newly discovered hormones called prostaglandins which have a wide range of effects on many tissues: on smooth muscle contraction, blood pressure and the nervous and reproductive systems. Essential fatty acids are also involved in skin metabolism and may play a part in preventing degenerative changes in the white matter of the brain and thus in the prevention of disease like multiple sclerosis and pre-senile dementia, in which the nervous system goes wrong before the rest of the body.

What we are seeing more and more today is a rise in degenerative diseases of all kinds due to our taking a diet poor in essential nutrients and high in useless carbohydrate fuel, refined and contaminated with additives to the point where our enzyme systems are clogged and poisoned. Hence, in a large part, the strokes, coronaries, digestive disorder, brain damage and deterioration, and, of course, obesity which is nothing more than a result of presenting to the body unsuitable calorie-laden carbohydrate food in unwieldy amounts at frequent intervals.

I tried eating meat fat, and was nearly sick in the middle of a meal shared with my husband! I had to find a way round this problem as I was getting dangerously underweight.

I come from a family of professional cooks, and there came into my mind the oft-repeated phrase that pork fat is good for the skin. I remembered my grandmother and my aunts rendering down pork fat into dripping, and the family eating it on toast. Perhaps there was something in it after all.

I tried it, and it worked. I cut all the fat from the meat, and rendered it down to liquid fat. Then I cooked the meat in its own fat, so that the fat dripping was absorbed into the lean meat. The crispy bits of fat left, after the rendering, are quite different from jelly-like fat, and are pleasant to eat. Now, I find that this way of cooking meat is not only palatable, but highly desirable.

I also remembered the broth that my grandmother and aunts had made, and this became an important part of my diet. It is made by boiling marrow bones for many hours (eight or more hours) which produces a thickish broth that can be drunk at any time. It is incredibly nutritious. My grandmother, who was very poor, brought up seven healthy children on this broth and very little else by way of first class protein. So did her mother before her. The children survived.

Bones are very cheap. My grandmother used to pay a penny for a bag of bones. Nowadays you can get a bag of bones for nothing!

I used any bones of meat that I could eat, but always broke them so that the marrow fat came out. I also added lumps of pork skin and pig's trotters because pork fat is good for the skin. The nutritional level of this broth must be very high indeed. My skin was perfect again, I had boundless vitality and I never felt hungry. When I was eating a high vegetable diet I was constantly hungry and couldn't wait for the next meal. On a high meat and animal fat diet, with the broth to drink, I never felt hunger pains.

But what about the dietary implications? Surely it is not healthy to live on meat alone? What, for example, about the effect upon the heart and the circulation?

Tony said that such anxieties were unfounded. There are plenty of communities in the human race who live on meat and fat only, and they are perfectly healthy. In the nineteenth and twentieth centuries, explorers, mountaineers, and any group of Western people cut off from supplies of fresh food would carry and live off a food called pemmican, which is dried meat in animal fat, he told me. They would live on this exclusively for months, and remain perfectly healthy. He reminded me that I was having vitamin and mineral supplements in addition, which was more than the early explorers had – and they still remained healthy.

Spring was advancing in all her beauty. It was the loveliest spring I can ever remember, and my skin was perfect. Tony continued to monitor my progress and after about two months of a meat and water diet he suggested re-introducing some plant foods. He explained very carefully the theory and practice of re-introduction* and of rotation of foods.* (*See Part II: 'Guide to re-introduction of Foods' and 'Rotation Diet and Food Supplements').

Tony recommended that I should obtain Soda Bicarbonate and Potassium Bicarbonate before commencing re-introduction. Soda Bicarbonate is easy to obtain from a chemist. Potassium Bicarbonate is not. (However, one manufacturer is J M Loveridge plc, Southampton, telephone number 023 8022 8411. A chemist can obtain it from the company.) In the event of a bad reaction to a food, take a mixture of 2 teaspoons of Soda Bicarbonate and one teaspoon of Potassium Bicarbonate dissolved in water. Drink a lot of water afterwards (not tap water). Repeat the dose every four hours until symptoms disappear. A horrible taste, but effective .

Tony advised trying only rare foods, that I had not eaten before. I obtained yams, sweet potatoes, cocoa root, cassava, mouli, oriental leaves, sago, tapioca, buckwheat.

At first all went well. I could eat and enjoy all these foods with no bad reaction, but after a few weeks the pattern changed and I had to accept total failure. One by one all these rare foods, which at first were tolerated well, a few weeks later precipitated a violent reaction – my skin flared up, and the maddening itch started all over again. The Soda/Potassium Bicarbonate mixture taken four-hourly reduced the reaction to the minimum – it is a very effective remedy.

Alarming and unexpected things were happening in other ways also. As well as the skin reaction I felt strangely unwell each time, a most curious feeling. I thought at first that I was imagining it, but it happened repeatedly. It was mostly profound lethargy, with a dull headache, heavy limbs, somewhat impaired vision and an inability to think clearly. The reaction was alarming, and I was beginning to dread the headache and lethargy almost as much as the itching.

I saw Tony again. He told me that the first time of eating a new food will not provoke a reaction – but it would have sensitized me. On subsequently eating the same food, the sensitization would cause a flare-up.

I asked him why I should feel so ill. It had not happened before.

He explained that allergies shift and change all the time. An allergic reaction to something will clear up unexpectedly, or a new allergy will develop for no known reason. Symptoms can likewise vary in a bewildering manner. Many different illnesses, both mental and physical can be caused by allergies to foods. The cause and symptoms in any one person can change all the time.

We agreed that there was no chance of me being able to re-introduce new foods, and that I must remain on a meat and water diet until I saw Professor Brostoff. My skin and my general health remained perfect, during the three months of waiting.

I saw Professor Jonathan Brostoff at the Middlesex Hospital, London in June 1995. He was impressed that severe eczema had been cured by diet alone, but told me that I needed a more mixed diet, because new allergies could develop to meat, and then I would have nothing to eat. He advised that I should be desensitized, and recommended enzyme potentiated desensitization (EPD), which is a form of immunotherapy.

⌘

Definition and diagnosis of food allergy and intolerance. Testing for food allergy and intolerance. Favourite foods and masked food allergy.

PART II

THE HIDDEN CAUSE?

PREFACE

Allergy or Intolerance?

A word must be said about the difference between *food allergy* and *food intolerance*. Most lay people find the medical terminology very confusing.

Food allergy is an acute, immediate reaction to an allergen. In extreme cases, such as peanut allergy, it can lead to anaphylactic shock or death.

Food intolerance is less acute, non-immediate, is not obvious and is not life threatening. It can, however, cause many chronic and debilitating diseases.

People who suffer from eczema will suffer from *food intolerance* and not *food allergy* in the strict medical sense of the words. Why then do I call the book *Eczema and Food Allergy* and use the word *allergy* when I know it to be wrong?

The simple answer is the use of language. An *allergy* is a noun, with a clear meaning in the minds of most people. *Intolerance* is not. You can use the adjective *allergic* and talk about an *allergic person*, and most people will understand you. But if you say an *intolerant person* it means something quite different.

Allergy can be made neatly into another noun, *an allergen*, meaning a substance which creates an *allergic* reaction in some people. This leads to the adjective *allergenic* - as in "Dust is very *allergenic*". But could the writer say "Dust is an *intolerogen* causing an *intolerogenic* reaction in an *intolerable* person"?

Of course not.

Chapter 3

THE HIDDEN CAUSE

Are you food allergic? Is it the hidden cause of your eczema? Think of food allergy as an iceberg, the greater part of which is hidden under the surface of the water.

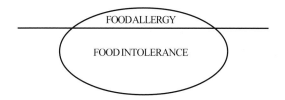

Food Allergy (gives a **positive** reaction to allergy tests).

This is an obvious condition. Violent reaction to food occurs within minutes. The condition is recognised by the medical profession, and doctors and dieticians know how to treat it.

Hidden Food Allergy or Intolerance (usually gives a **negative** reaction to tests).

(NOTE: Hidden food allergy, masked food allergy, delayed food allergy, non-immediate food allergy, and food intolerance all mean the same thing. Medical terminology can get very confusing!)

Hidden food allergy, or intolerance, is well and truly hidden and accounts for the greater part of the iceberg. Usually many hidden food allergies exist in one person, and co-exist with inhaled or contact allergies.

1   The reaction to food is not obvious.
2   The reaction may take days to develop.
3   Hidden food allergies can cause illness in all systems of
    the body.
4   These illnesses can shift and change over the years.
5   The hidden allergies can also change.
6   Usually the sufferer is unaware of the cause of the illness.
7   Hidden food allergy (intolerance) is widespread in the
    population.
8   There is a link to gut fermentation (candida).
9   There is also a link to chemical sensitivity.

Most people with eczema do not have an immediate food allergy, but may well have a hidden food allergy (intolerance). If you go to your doctor with this suggestion, he or she may suggest a skin test or patch test. The result will probably be negative. Hidden food allergy has not been accurately revealed by any tests that I have heard of, in spite of claims to the contrary. The only way to reveal a hidden food intolerance in my experience is an elimination diet.

Many people spend a small fortune on commercial "tests" which claim to prove which foods individual people are allergic to. These tests may show up some allergies or intolerances, but none of them are wholly reliable.

If you, the reader, suspect food allergies but are not sure, quicker, more accurate and much cheaper than any tests would be a positive answer to several of the following questions:

➤   Do you know of any member of your family who was or is food allergic? There is a strong genetic and hereditary tendency amongst blood relatives.

➤   Have you ever been ill, not eaten for a few days, and found your eczema cleared significantly, only to return once you started eating again?

➢ Does the skin around your mouth ever go red and itchy, or your lips and tongue swell after eating certain foods?

➢ Do you have repeated mouth ulcers?

➢ Do you have abdominal discomfort or swelling after eating certain foods?

➢ Do you know from experience that certain foods make your skin worse? Such as nuts, fish especially shellfish or crustacea, curry, or very spicy foods, fruit, alcohol?

➢ Would you say that you are addicted to any type of food, and think you couldn't live without it? This could indicate a masked food allergy.

➢ Are you a vegetarian or a "health food" addict? Many plant foods and "health foods" are highly allergenic.

➢ Do you eat a lot of convenience foods? Commercially prepared foods usually contain a lot of chemical additives. You might be chemically sensitive. Tap water contains a lot of chemicals. Have you ever suspected it?

➢ Does your skin flare up if you take aspirin, Codeine, Anadin, cough or throat mixtures, or similar patent medicines? Do you know of any drug allergy?

➢ Does alcohol cause a flare-up?

If you answer "yes" to several of these questions, there is a high chance that food allergy is at least a part of the cause of your eczema, in which case an elimination dict is well worth trying.

Favourite foods

The hardest thing to accept about food allergy is that it will always be the foods that you most enjoy, and eat most frequently, to which you are most allergic. It is somehow linked to addiction. This phenomena has been noted by every allergy specialist. If you think you cannot do without a certain food, and feel better (in the short term) for eating it, you can be 90% sure that it is among the chief causes of your eczema.

Why favourite foods are the most allergenic, and why you have not noticed it before is interesting. It is called the *hidden* or *masked allergy.*

The effect is rather like smoking or alcohol addiction. The first cigarette seems unpleasant to you, but for some reason you have another, and then another. Very soon you cannot do without it. Your body seems to need the nicotine. You feel withdrawal symptoms if you cannot have a smoke, and the nicotine level in your body drops. You begin to feel a craving for the next cigarette, and it can seem intolerable if you are not able to get one. When you do get one, the first inhalation for the smoker seems blissful, as the nicotine enters the bloodstream. The body relaxes, and a feeling of well-being ensues. This pattern is invariable, even though all the time the nicotine is poisoning you and in some people (not all) will eventually cause health problems.

The pattern is the same with food addictions. The body seems to crave the very thing that is doing it the most harm. So you eat it every day, often two or three times a day. It is therefore always present in your digestive system and in your bloodstream. If you have to do without it for any length of time you begin to long for it. When you eventually get the food, it seems to do you good, producing a true feeling of comfort and well-being. It is because the food is always present in your body that you are unaware of the trouble it is causing.

If you are going to pursue the elimination diet for the cause and cure of your eczema, you will almost certainly have to give up all your favourites, at least during the first phase of the diet. (You may be able to re-introduce some of them later.) If you do not think you have the will-power to do this, perhaps it is better for you to live with the eczema. The decision will depend upon the severity of the eczema, and the effect it has upon your life.

From personal experience I can say that following a strict elimination diet was the hardest thing I have ever done in my life.

⌘

Chapter 4

OTHER CAUSES OF ECZEMA

The four ways in which allergens enter the body. The dangers of chemical and drug allergy. Fungal disbiosis of the gut.

Medical teaching states that the classical allergic diseases are asthma, eczema, dermatitis, urticaria, hives, hay fever and rhinitis.

Atopic eczema is an allergic disease. 'Atopic' means 'A tendency to develop allergies.' From the Greek it also means 'Of no fixed place', and there is nothing fixed or certain about allergies or allergic diseases.

Food is not the only cause of eczema. There are many other causes, which will be considered below.

An allergic reaction can be triggered by:

1. **CONTACT** - Animals especially cats, birds, grass, pollens, dust, latex rubber, surgical sticking plasters.

Anything touching the skin.

2. **INJECTIONS** - Wasp or bee stings, mosquito bites etc., drugs.

Anything penetrating the skin.

3. **INHALATION** - Animal dander, perfumes, vapours from paints, sprays, house dust mite, fumes from vehicles, cleaning products.

Anything inhaled into the lungs.

4. **INGESTION** - Food, drinks, drugs, food additives and chemical residue on food.

Anything entering the alimentary tract.

Atopic people are usually sensitive to more than one type of allergen, because they are all inter-related and all can trigger each other off.

I will enlarge upon each, in turn:

CONTACT ALLERGENS

Contact dermatitis can be caused by something touching the skin, causing a local reaction. The term is quite frequently used to mean atopic eczema (and vice versa), which is not surprising as the two conditions overlap, and sometimes cannot be separated for diagnostic purposes.

Contact dermatitis occurs shortly after contact with the allergen, and the cause is usually known. Examples would be a skin rash due to contact with a metal zip; itchy skin due to a woollen jumper; a reaction to certain types of make-up or skin creams; local reaction to sticky plaster, or proximity to a cat. Cats are a major allergenic cause of asthma and eczema.

Contact dermatitis can also be less obvious and less easily recognised, such as a generalised rash due to cats or sensitivity to the house dust mite; autumnal rash due to mould spores (often not recognised); springtime rash due to pollens. These examples can overlap with eczema.

I do not underestimate the importance of contact allergens, but others have dealt with the subject. It usually responds well to a mild hydrocortisone cream, given for a limited period.

The National Eczema Society offers help and advice about the avoidance of contact allergens. Eczema can improve dramatically if you follow the Society's advice about the control of the house dust mite. The dust mite is a major cause of atopic asthma and eczema, and you need to clear your home of it, as far as possible. Animals in a home create dust and dander for the house dust mite to breed in.

Contact to many chemicals causes dermatitis. I think of soaps and detergents, fabric softeners, etc. Change to non-chemical cleaning substances will often clear the dermatitis. But, if the offending substances are repeatedly used, the dermatitis can progress to eczema, which will not clear.

Contact with latex rubber is a fast growing allergic condition with very serious consequences. It is thought to have originated with the widespread use of cheap latex gloves in hospitals. My own theory is that many newborn babies are sensitised at birth by latex gloves worn by midwives and doctors, (See *Neo-natal Sensitisation to Latex**.) Latex allergy can cause eczema and the only known treatment is total avoidance. This is a big subject outside the scope of this book, but if a young child appears to develop a rash around the mouth after (for example) sucking a rubber toy, it could well be due to latex allergy. The Latex Allergy Support Group can help and advise.

*Available from Action Against Allergy, see Useful Addresses.

INJECTED ALLERGENS AND DRUG ALLERGIES

Wasp and bee stings, jelly fish stings, and other insect bites are forms of injected allergens. They can cause an acute reaction, but I have never heard that they can cause eczema.

I firmly believe that drugs, taken orally or injected, can be and are a frequent cause of many allergic diseases, including eczema. Most drugs are chemically derived and many people are acutely chemically sensitive. The possibility of a drug or medicine provoking an allergenic reaction in your body, causing eczema, should not be overlooked.

I have a very old copy of Conybeare's *Textbook of Medicine 1943* (first edition 1929). It states in the section on eczema that drugs can provoke erythmatous rashes. The textbook lists some of the drugs then in use, which were known to cause this problem: opium, mercury, quinine, copaiba, phenolphthaline, the iodides and bromides, salicylates, digitalis, belladonna.

Consider how relatively few drugs were in use fifty to one hundred years ago, yet many were known to cause skin problems. Compare this in your mind with the hundreds of thousands of sophisticated chemical drugs that are used today. Then consider, if it was a recognised medical fact in those days that drugs caused skin troubles, how much more relevant it will be today. Will not skin problems be multiplied proportionately to the multiplication of drugs prescribed or bought?

Yet I do not know that drugs are ever considered as a cause of atopic eczema. The incidence of eczema and asthma is rising, and the established medical world does not know why. I have yet to meet a dermatologist or any other conventionally trained doctor, for that matter, who would say that drugs can cause allergic diseases. Allergy specialists certainly say so but they still lack recognition by many of their medical peers, and their voices go largely unheeded.

The worst thing about drug allergy is that it can trigger off allergic or intolerant reactions to other things months or even years later, so the link is not always obvious. Also, there is no telling what a cocktail of drugs, taken over a long period, will do to the body. There could be a cumulative reaction.

It is not surprising that the modern phenomenon of the increased incidence of allergic diseases (approaching epidemic proportions) receives so little research. The multi-national pharmaceutical companies, who virtually control medical research, would be seriously embarrassed if it were proved that their drugs were a major cause of allergic disease. We are talking about billions of pounds of vested interest here, and I see no way out of it.

My only advice to any atopic person is to be very wary of taking any prescribed drug or patent medicine, and particularly of giving them to children whose immune system is underdeveloped.

INHALED ALLERGENS

These are things breathed into the lungs. They are thought to cause asthma and hay fever, more than eczema. However, I am not sure that I believe this. I think that the role of inhaled allergens in the cause of eczema is just as hidden as is the role of food allergy.

There are two types of inhaled allergens:

> Natural allergens

> Chemical allergens

Natural Inhaled Allergens

These are natural particles in the air, like pollens, grass, animal hair and dander. These things have been known for centuries to cause hay fever or wheezing in some people. They are usually seasonal, and people just have to avoid them. Asthma UK offers reliable advice on identifying and avoiding natural inhaled allergens.

Chemical Inhaled Allergens

The inhalation of chemicals from fumes, perfumes, spray vapours etc. is much more omnipresent than we think. The air we breath is most foully polluted. You only have to enter the "household cleaning" area of a supermarket to be knocked sideways by the stench. The perfume department of a big store not only smells like a whore-house, but the fumes can cause instant asthma. Imagine living next to a copy shop or a dry cleaning shop – it would be enough to give any baby asthma or eczema. High level spraying of farm land spreads chemicals far and wide. Council authorities spray poisonous chemicals in public places, including children's playgrounds, to kill the weeds. These are only a few examples. When inhaled these chemicals enter the blood stream, and we do not know the damage they cause.

It is now estimated that over 4 million chemical substances are present in the atmosphere. The toxicity to mammalian life has not been adequately tested either singly or in combination.

You are not going to be able to get away from chemicals in the environment. What you *can* do though is to restrict to the minimum those in your home.

Do not underestimate the importance of this. Recent study has shown that chemical products in our homes, particularly hermetically sealed houses, are a significant cause of the increase of allergic diseases during the last forty years.

This is a list of some of the domestic chemicals that are known to cause allergic reactions:

o   Many cleaning substances, especially perfumed ones
o   Detergents, most washing powders
o   Fabric softeners
o   Air fresheners and deodorisers
o   Gas fumes, including central heating
o   Domestic and garden pesticides
o   Many cosmetics and hair preparations
o   Perfumes, after-shave, body sprays, deodorants
o   Carpets
o   Fire resistant fabrics
o   Plastics, formaldehyde
o   Glues and solvents
o   Synthetically made, fitted furniture
o   Paints, varnishes, vinyl wallpaper
o   Insulating materials
o   The interior of a new car
o   Glossy magazines
o   Dry cleaning of clothes
o   Synthetic fabrics and 'conditioned' clothes
o   Latex rubber

This is not intended as a complete list. There are many others! I seriously advise mothers of young children with asthma or eczema to eliminate as far as possible inhaled chemical allergens from the home. In my opinion asthma and eczema are a direct consequence of a chemically polluted home.

As I walk around towns and cities and villages, I see thousands of young women pushing tiny babies in smart little prams. They are very low, about the level of car or lorry exhaust fumes, and the baby faces forwards inhaling the fumes. This seems to be terribly dangerous, and I advise any mother who has a history of atopy in the family, to acquire a high pram, away from the fumes, to protect her baby.

On the subject of babies – perfumes these days are all made from chemicals. The days when perfume was made from flowers are long since past. Any woman who wears perfume and breast feeds a baby is forcing the child to inhale an unknown quantity of unnamed chemicals

INGESTED ALLERGENS

This is the main subject of this book, and under this heading I would like to talk about chemical additives in foods, of which there are now over 4000, and the number is growing all the time. In addition there is chemical residue left on food from farming, storing and manufacture.

Nobody knows the effects they have on the human body. Immediate effects are tested for, and if any are found to be harmful the chemical is banned. However, the accumulated effects of chemicals taken into the body over many hears cannot be monitored, nor can chemicals reacting with each other be monitored. Additionally, certain chemicals are declared to be "safe" in some countries, but banned as "unsafe" in other countries.

The subject of fungal disbiosis (candida) can be considered in this context, because an excess of chemicals in the gut is thought to be one of the causes of widespread fungal disbiosis in the population. Fungal spores can penetrate the gut wall causing a "leaky gut", which some doctors say is at the root of all food allergy. It is a serious condition requiring medical treatment. The British Society for Ecological Medicine (BSEM) can advise.

As though all this were not enough, there is also the possibility of heavy metals in the body causing a breakdown of immune function. Mercury fillings in teeth are the most common source, and the British Society for Mercury Free Dentistry* can advise.

So you can see why with all these different sorts of allergenic triggers, all of them capable of cross-reacting with each other, it is so difficult to get to the root of eczema.

*See Useful Addresses

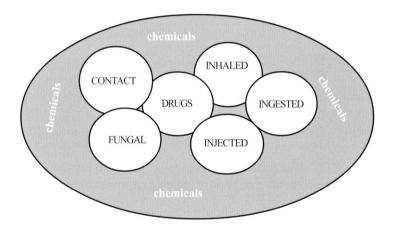

⌘

Chapter 5

FOOD ALLERGY

A challenge to conventional thinking about an elimination diet, with a warning about the difficulties and dangers

This book concentrates on *food allergy*, which is a sadly neglected cause of many illnesses.

I have had letters from all over the country from people who think their eczema is due to food, but their doctors cannot help them.

However, there are a few allergy specialists in the country (guidance in finding one is given at the end of this book) and if you can possibly find one, this would be by far your best course of action. An elimination diet and re-introduction of foods is very complex, full of unforeseen difficulties and pitfalls, and nothing can replace one-to-one consultation with a specialist. However, with very few exceptions, such specialist treatment is not available on the NHS, and consequently you may have to pay private medical fees.

If you cannot find a private allergy specialist, have no medical insurance and cannot afford private treatment, your only course will be to follow an elimination diet on your own, which is why I have written this book. It is a step by step guide to help you to identify and eliminate allergenic foods from your diet and to help you understand the nature of your atopy.

However, I must stress that the book *is not intended* for the treatment of children or pregnant women, for whom specialist treatment is mandatory.

It can be very dangerous to try an elimination diet on a child without expert help. After a period of abstinence there is an increased sensitivity to an allergenic substance. A child can react with anaphylactic shock, which can be fatal.

You will find that the diet, and the management of it, is very strict indeed, even extreme. This is intentional. Both asthma and eczema are notoriously hard to treat, by any means, including diet. In fact, both diseases are said to be incurable. If you are going to find your food allergies and intolerances, you are going to have to work at it. There is no point in approaching it in a half-hearted way.

Most adults who have tried some sort of elimination diet for the treatment of eczema have reported that it does not work. This may be why the medical profession states that there is little or no link between eczema and food.

I challenge this assumption. If the elimination diet has not worked, it will be for one or more of a number of reasons.

1. The diet is wrong or wrongly understood.

2. The need for TOTAL elimination (not just partial) has not been understood.

3. The re-introduction phase has been mishandled.

4. Rotation of foods, after re-introduction, has been ignored.

5. The immune system is so disordered by years of steroid treatments that the body cannot respond to anything.

6. Fungal disbiosis of the gut has not been considered.

7. Other allergenic triggers have not been considered.

⌘

Chapter 6

INFORM YOUR DOCTOR

Concerning the advisability of obtaining medical support for an elimination diet

You should inform your doctor if you intend seriously to try an elimination diet and try to enlist his interest and support. Many doctors will be very sceptical and will tell you that it will not work and that you will be wasting your time and energy. Do not believe it. Properly conducted, an elimination diet will work, and if it does not there will be good and identifiable reasons.

Your doctor may suggest a RAST test. This is the best of the medical tests available on the NHS. If he does, I suggest you should be tested for:

Milk, eggs, wheat, yeast, potato, soya.

Don't be surprised if the report is negative to everything. The RAST is notorious for coming up with false negatives. It merely means that you are not actually allergic to these things, by the true definition of the word. You may well be intolerant of them and this will not be revealed by the test.

Your doctor may advise you to take hypo-allergenic vitamin and mineral supplements. These are available on prescription through the NHS. The main thing is that you must **not** take supplements bought off the shelf from chemists and health food shops. These will be made from many of the things that you will have to eliminate initially, such as yeast, soya, wheat, maize, fish oils, fruits. They will also contain many additives that you must eliminate, such as colouring and flavouring.

You will have to come off all but life-saving drugs during the elimination phase of the diet. You might be allergic to the drug without knowing it. Apart from the drug itself, the tablet will be made up in a starch base (which holds the tablet together), usually derived from maize, wheat, soya, potato, all of which you must eliminate. Linctuses are made from sugars, usually corn/maize sugar and most of these preparations contain colourings or flavourings. All must be eliminated.

If your eczema is very severe and you are on steroid tablets you cannot possibly stop taking them. Your doctor must be involved here. If you respond well to the diet you will be able to reduce the steroids over a period of time, but you cannot do this alone and must have medical direction.

Steroid creams are easier to reduce and this can be done either by using a weaker strength cream or by progressively reducing the quantity and frequency of application. It is a question of titrating the amount and strength of the cream against the improvement resulting from the diet, and your doctor needs to be involved.

You may have a candida or fungal infestation of the gut and/or the skin. Candida is not often considered as a cause of eczema but it can be, and frequently is. In fact, a leading allergy specialist has told me that in his experience candidiasis so frequently accompanies food allergies that he now includes anti-fungal treatment in all his dietary and desensitising treatments. You could discuss the possibility with your doctor and ask him if he would prescribe a course of anti-fungal treatment to be taken *at the same time* as a complete elimination of all sugars and yeasts and a substantial reduction of starches and carbohydrates.

Your next step is to learn as much as you possibly can about allergies, and food allergies in particular. The more you know about the subject the better you will be able to help yourself. I can particularly recommend Brostoff and Gamlin's *The Complete Guide to Food Allergy and Intolerance*.

Many other books are available but you must be selective. You can get helpful advice from Merton Books a mail order supplier which specialises in books to help with special diets. *(See Useful Addresses.)*

Chapter 7

UNDERSTANDING THE DIET

The two golden rules for a successful elimination diet.
The need for attention to detail.

Understanding the diet is vitally important. I am quite sure that most elimination diets fail because they are imperfectly understood. The patient and his or her doctor then concludes that food allergy is not the cause of the eczema, when all the time it is.

The diet falls into two phases:

Elimination

Re-introduction.

With eczema, the diet, if properly conducted, will take a minimum of three to four weeks to be effective. This is the length of time it takes for the skin to renew itself. If the eczema is very severe or of long standing and the skin is very thickened with much scarring from scratching it will take longer to heal. However, if allergenic foods have been eliminated, the eczema will not be erupting from beneath the skin surface all the time and the itching will get progressively less, and the skin will have a chance to heal.

The first three to four weeks are the crucial time for eczema sufferers, when you must understand exactly what you are doing, and why, and be very careful indeed about the details given in the following pages.

During the first week you may experience withdrawal symptoms. These can take many forms: you may feel ill and sick; dizzy and shaky; you may feel light-headed and lacking in concentration; you may feel lethargic and sluggish with a nasty headache. All these strange reactions are signs that a "masked" food allergy is being unmasked. You will almost certainly feel a craving for your favourite foods. But whatever you do, don't give in to this craving. If you do, you will go right back to square one. Withdrawal symptoms go after about a week.

On the other hand, you may experience no withdrawal symptoms at all. In fact, quite the opposite – you may feel wonderful on the restricted diet. There is no telling. Everyone is different.

From the beginning you must keep a diary of exactly what you eat. A blank exercise book is best, recording foods eaten on the left hand side and reactions or general condition on the right.

If you understand and apply the two golden rules of an elimination diet, you enhance your chances of success. If you fail to understand their importance and are slack about them you are unlikely to succeed.

The golden rules are:

1. All potentially allergenic foods must be eliminated at the same time.

2. The tiniest particle of an allergenic food can cause an allergic reaction.

Let me enlarge on this.

Everything must be eliminated at once.

People with severe atopic eczema, usually, are not just intolerant of one or two things. They react to many different substances in their diet. There is no point at all in eliminating only some of the allergenic foods. All the possible suspects must go at once, leaving only enough food to keep the body healthy.

The tiniest particle of an allergenic food can cause an allergic reaction.

This may seem hard to believe, but it is a fact that you will have to accept. Tiny, even microscopic, particles of an offending food can have a very nasty effect.

I firmly believe that failure to understand these two points is the reason for the failure of many attempted elimination diets. If foods are incompletely avoided not only will the symptoms fail to clear, but challenge testing to establish intolerance may be invalidated because of the masking of the response, i.e. the tiny amount still in the bloodstream may "protect" the individual from flare up symptoms on re-introduction.

Elimination has to be total. There can be no compromise at all. No bending of the rules, or secret lapses because no-one is looking. No tiny glass of something, because everyone else is having it. If you do this it will set you back five days, the time it takes to clear the bowel of residue. If you do it every day you might as well abandon the diet altogether.

Sublingual absorption must be considered here. Anything is absorbed into the bloodstream more quickly and effectively from under the tongue than from the stomach, where it is mixed with gastric juices. Furthermore, sublingual absorption by-passes the liver. Therefore do not suck anything at all whilst you are on the diet. Do not lick stamps or envelopes. Do not lick your fingers if they get prohibited food on them, such as happens if you are cooking for others, or if you are eating with children. Do not sample a food you are cooking for others to see if it has the right flavour or if it is done. You will be absorbing sublingually all sorts of things that will go straight into your bloodstream, and if you are allergic to them they may cause your eczema to flare up and set you back five days in your diet.

Toothpaste is a prime example of sublingual absorption. These contain unknown amounts of colourings, flavourings, bleaches, gels, in addition to the food starch base, all of which will be absorbed into your bloodstream. Do not touch them. Use a mixture of bicarbonate of soda and sea salt. Throw away your old toothbrush which will be contaminated. Do not use mouthwashes or suck mouth fresheners. Never chew gum.

However careful you are, accidents will always happen and cooking will be the main source of such accidents. It is best, as least during the elimination stage, if all your food and cooking is kept quite separate from others. A trace of food left in a saucepan or on a spoon would contaminate your food. Do not use mugs that have been stained brown from tea or coffee. You will be ingesting molecules of tannin or caffeine. You must be scrupulous about washing up and strict about rinsing things. Traces of detergent left on crockery or cutlery would be ingested. Soda is safer to use. No-one with eczema who has any sense would put their hands into a bowl of detergent water. We all wear gloves. But latex rubber is very allergenic and can inflame the skin. Wear instead PVC cotton-lined gloves.

Take care to avoid contamination of your food. A few crumbs from someone else's bread falling into your food could cause a nasty flare up for you, and you would probably be unaware of the cause of the flare up. It is best if your food is kept on the top shelf of the fridge or larder so that things cannot fall into it.

You will not be able to take bits of food from a general dish cooked for other people because molecules of foods that you are eliminating will have penetrated the whole dish. I think of stews or casseroles as an example. A stew is nearly always thickened with flour or cornflour, molecules of which will have penetrated the meat and vegetables, so you cannot eat them.

Some people react to the chemical contaminants in tap water. To avoid this it is better that you should drink only bottled water from a *reputable* natural spring. (Unfortunately, some bottled waters have been shown to be more contaminated than tap water.) If you do this you will not only have to drink bottled water but all vegetables will have to be cooked in it during the elimination phase. You can steam vegetables, using tap water. Do not use a microwave, because the radiated food might harm you.

All these finicky details are time-consuming and tiresome, but they must be observed to the letter if the elimination diet is to be effective.

You must know exactly what goes into your mouth at all times in order to isolate allergies.

If you cook for yourself and understand the requirements, and are very careful, you increase considerably the chance of a successful outcome. But if someone else cooks for you it can be more difficult and can lead to strained relationships. It has to be a very devoted wife/mother/partner who will remember and observe all the necessary details of the diet. If she cannot be trusted to do so it would be better if you took over cooking for yourself in order that you can be confident of the result of your dietary test. Cooking is important, because cooked food is less allergenic than uncooked food.

Eating away from home is difficult and you will have to take your food with you, but most people are very understanding, I find. It is best to plan the elimination phase of the diet to coincide with a time when you do not have to eat away from home. Once you are well into the re-introduction phase it becomes easier.

If you smoke you must give it up whilst on an elimination diet. Smoking is known to trigger off allergic problems and must be eliminated along with all the other potentially allergenic foods.

As a communicant Christian I know that it is not possible to take the bread and wine at communion. The wheat from the bread will be absorbed sublingually and so will the fruit juices, the yeasts and the sugar from the wine. Suggestion: pre-arrange with the priest to give you a blessing.

Chemical Sensitivity

If you suspect that you are acutely sensitive to chemicals, it would be worth testing this before starting an elimination diet.

You would need to buy only organically grown fresh foods for three to four weeks and have *nothing else at all* during that time. No commercially prepared foods of any sort, even if the packet label says it is "organic". Drink only bottled water from a reputable

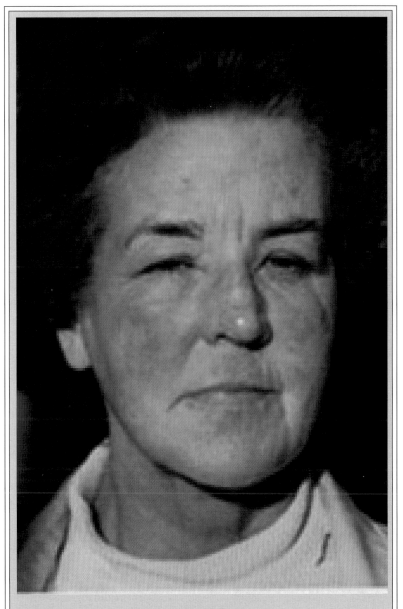

This photograph and those overleaf were taken in December 1994, approximately six months after the worst stage of which I have no photographic record.

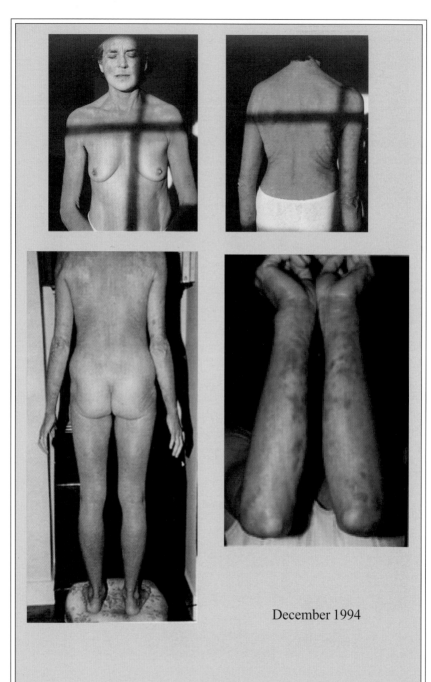

December 1994

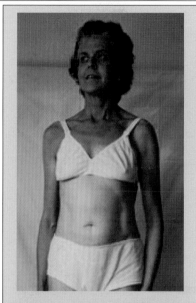
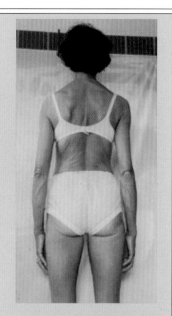
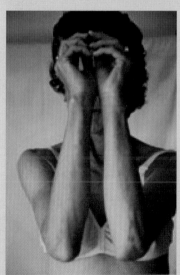
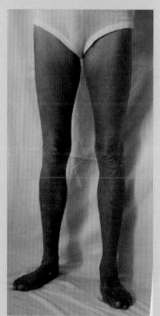

March 1995

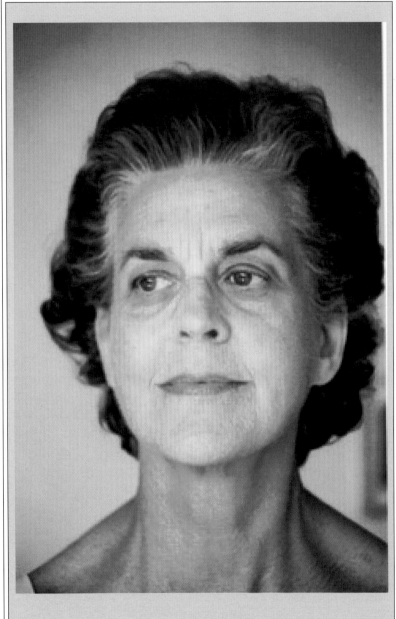
The author in March 1995

spring. No tea, coffee, cocoa, coffee substitutes, herb tea, etc., because the drying processes of such beverages are chemical (frequently sulphur dioxide); no dried foods of any sort for the same reason. No alcohol, it is full of unnamed additives.

However, I tried organically grown foods only for three weeks and it made no difference at all to my skin. I understand this to be the general experience. It is paradoxical but it seems to be something in the nature of the food itself that causes the trouble. On the other hand, the E-range of food additives could cause a flare up of my skin within half an hour of eating.

Nickel Sensitivity

Some people are nickel sensitive. If you are it can be difficult because practically all metal kitchen equipment, including cutlery, contains nickel. To test the possibility wear a pair of jeans with a cheap nickel zip over the abdomen for a day. If your skin flares up you are nickel sensitive.

No research (or very little) has been done on this so I am skating on thin ice, but it seems to me that if nickel applied externally will provoke an allergenic reaction, molecules of nickel taken internally will cause as much, or more trouble. To test this you would have to use only wooden, pyrex or earthenware cooking equipment and cutlery for three to four weeks. I have had letters from people who tell me that by eliminating all nickel cooking equipment they have improved their eczema by 80 - 90%.

Amalgam in the Teeth

Do not have dental treatment whilst on an elimination diet. The injections, the antiseptics, the latex gloves dentists wear, could cause a flare up. Apart from that, the mercury in amalgam fillings is a serious poison which has made a lot of people very ill. For advice on this matter see addresses at the end of the book.

⌘

Chapter 8

VEGETARIANS

I must address a special section to vegetarians with whom I have a special sympathy, because I had been a vegetarian all my life, from earliest childhood onwards, until severe eczema turned my life upside down.

If you seriously want to search for food allergies as the possible cause of your eczema for one reason or another (which will be explained later) you will have to give up everything but meat and vegetables and a limited amount of carbohydrate. All foods containing second-class protein will have to be set aside for diagnostic purposes.

Historically there are only two sources of food for man – animal flesh and edible plants. Of these, the animal meats are the *least* troublesome and the plant foods the *most* troublesome (although eggs and milk are highly allergenic).

It has now been shown that there are natural chemical compounds running throughout the entire plant family to which some people, the hypersensitive among us, are allergic or intolerant. This theory is currently being researched in America and Europe. It is the only possible theory, which would explain why so many people are allergic to so many plants – inhaled, contact or foods. Less commonly, does man show an intolerance to meats.

Vegetarians love plant foods and live on them exclusively. We are assured by all the modern food specialists that the most healthy foods are the plant foods, particularly the "wholemeal" types. Then why should they be poorly tolerated by some people?

"Health foods" are not the same as "allergenic" foods. For the majority of the population I am quite sure that the healthy plant foods are the best and the most health-giving. But I am not addressing the majority of the population. I am writing for the minority who are hypersensitive, for the larger number of whom the plant foods will be the most troublesome.

Most plants contain poisons, developed by natural selection to protect the plant and deter animals or insects from eating them. Now, it may seem a bit far fetched to suggest that you or I are like the panda or the antelope who goes out selecting the plants that it can eat, who knows from inherited instinct what it cannot eat. However we, the human species, are animals and some among us, the atopic, will not be able to tolerate certain plant foods. This will differ from person to person because allergies always do, but the fact must be accepted that it will usually be plants that cause the greatest trouble for the hypersensitive person.

Just consider for a moment what a sniff of pollen does to those who suffer from hay fever or asthma. Consider what touching stinging nettles will do to you. Many plants in the countryside will aggravate most cases of eczema. If these things are true, it is not so hard to realise that actually eating plants, taking them into your body, will cause an allergic reaction in some people. The great poisoners of history have all be experts in plant knowledge and what plant juices will kill, and in what proportions to administer them.

The animal flesh that human beings eat is that of herbivores. We do not regularly eat the flesh of carnivorous animals. The herbivores have already eaten the plants and their systems have already detoxified the chemical components in the plants that are a source of allergenic reactions for atopic people. If we eat the flesh of these animals, we consume the nutrients and vitamins of the plants that have gone into building the body of the animal, but not the chemical compounds of the plants themselves.

I was discussing this with a leading allergy specialist who said: "No-one who is atopic can afford to be vegetarian."

I have no doubt that this will seem nauseating to the vegetarian reader, and I sympathise. I can only suggest that you should try, for a limited period of three weeks, the meat diet suggested and see what happens to your skin.

However, vegetarianism is a deeply held conviction, often with religious connotations, and you may be unable to change. My only practical suggestion is that you could ask your doctor to have a RAST test done for you, testing your favourite plant foods: wheatgerm, oats, nuts, beans and lentils, fruits, honey, seeds, rice, potatoes, dried fruits and (unless you are vegan) milk, cheese, yoghurt and eggs. If the RAST comes up positive though you can be reasonable sure that vegetarianism is a significant cause of your eczema.

If you really cannot eat meat and are plant sensitive there may be a way round this through desensitisation.

About 40 years ago I was a member of a religious organisation and vegetarianism was an obligation. I noticed that a large proportion of the older vegans (not the young ones) seemed to have nasty skin diseases. I knew nothing about eczema and had never heard of food allergies, but it stuck in my mind.

⌘

PART III

THE ELIMINATION DIET

Chapter 9

THE GOLDEN RULES

**Fasting – a thirty foods diet – a three foods diet.
The need for self-control on a very strict diet.**

To clear the alimentary tract of allergens is the aim. Therefore, if you can fast altogether for two, three or four days you will benefit.

Fasting for limited periods is widely practised in the Orient and it is regarded as beneficial to the health of mind and body. In modern Western culture the idea of abstaining from food for any length of time is anathema. But our obsessive eating habits are harmful.

It is necessary to drink, and you will find that warm water, taken at blood temperature, to which a teaspoonful of glycerine has been added, will allay hunger pangs. Glycerine is sweet, and is a bi-product of animal fat.

After fasting, there is a choice between two different diets:

The first involves about thirty different foods.

The second, only three different foods.

Which ever you choose, you must remember the golden rules.

1. ALL POTENTIALLY ALLERGENIC FOODS MUST BE ELIMINATED AT THE SAME TIME.

2. THE TINIEST PARTICLE OF AN ALLERGENIC FOOD CAN CAUSE A SEVERE REACTION.

Remember also:

➤ It takes 4-5 days for the bowel to be cleared of food residue.
➤ It takes 3-4 weeks for the skin to renew itself.

Let me start with the wider diet, which will probably be sufficient if your eczema is of mild or moderate severity.

THIRTY FOODS DIET

You will need to keep a diary.

All foods must be fresh, and it is preferable if they are organically grown, and the meat organically reared, because you may be chemically sensitive.

All foods must be cooked – cooking seems to reduce the allergenic properties in foods. Vegetables must be cooked in bottled water, or steamed. All cooking utensils must be scrupulously clean and rinsed because particles of other foods or detergent residue will be a contaminant. You must have no commercially prepared foods of any sort.

Whilst any foods can be allergenic to anyone, those suggested below are the least likely to be troublesome.

The foods you can take with reasonable safety are limited, and you will need at least three-four weeks on this diet before you see a significant improvement in your skin.

1. **Bottled spring water from a reputable source only for drinking and cooking**.

    No tea or coffee or any other stimulant drinks. *No* alcohol. *No* fruit juices.

2. **Meats**
    Lamb*, pork*, mutton*, rare meats, (if you can get them) venison, wild boar, buffalo, horse, kangaroo, ostrich, whale. NOT beef or veal. Ham or bacon*· Keep the liquid fat and the juices from the meat for gravy. (*No* commercial gravy powders; stamp marks on meat must be cut away because the dye is unknown.)

67

* Some people are sensitive to the regularly eaten meats, particularly pork. If you are, or suspect you are, do not eat them. Eat only rare meats or poultry or game.

3. **Poultry**
   Free range turkey, guinea fowl. Especially fatty birds like duck or goose, and eat the fat. Keep the juices for gravy. *NOT* chicken.

4. **Game**
   Wild rabbit, hare, pheasant, partridge, grouse, quail.

5 **Leafy vegetables – cooked**
   Cabbage, kale, spinach, red cabbage, Brussels, Brussel tops, cauliflower, broccoli, bean sprouts, artichokes, cooked celery (*not* raw celery). *NOT* pippy vegetables including peas and beans. *NOT* mushrooms or any fungal food.

6. **Root vegetables – peeled and cooked**
   Swede, carrot, parsnips**, turnips, sweet potatoes, cassava, yams, coco root, Chinese radish (mouli), celeriac (cooked), beetroot **. *NOT* Potatoes. *NOT* onions. *NOT* raw carrot.

7. **Salt**
   Coarse sea salt, with no "free-running" chemical added.

8. **Oils**
   Olive oil or sunflower oil for cooking (but not very much and *NOT* maize or nut oils or blended oils). It is better to use meat fat for cooking.

9. **Thickeners for gravy**
   Arrowroot, buckwheat flour, sago flour, tapioca (but not very much).

10. **No smoking**

11.   No sugars of any sort

12.   No uncooked foods.

**Beetroot and parsnip can be tricky. They have a high sugar content so be careful.

Carbohydrates
Carbohydrates have a tendency to cross-react with each other, even things from widely differing food families. It seems that one thing will trigger off an intolerance to another, or perhaps it is a build-up of any carbohydrates in the body that causes the trouble. There are some people who are intolerant of all carbohydrates, and if you are one such it would be advisable for you be desensitised.

If you cut out all bread, potatoes, rice, pasta, biscuits and cakes from your diet and rely solely on root vegetables for bulk, you will get hungry. It is not impossible to do so, but for four weeks it is difficult. My advice would be to take a *mixed grain* mixture of uncommonly eaten grains and seeds.

Do not include any of the commonly eaten grains at all.

Mixed Grains
Mix one part each of:
  Sago (small pearls)
  Tapioca
  Quinoa
  Alfalfa
  Buckwheat
  Millet
  Sunflower seed
  Linseed

Cooking time in water about 15-20 minutes. Add sea salt only and a little olive oil if you like.

This makes a thick rice/pasta type mixture. It is not wildly exciting but better than nothing. Do not add any flavourings. If you must have a sweet mix, add pork fat or glycerine. The advantage of the mix is that by taking such a small amount of each, the body will not develop a new intolerance to any one grain.

Bread substitute
It is possible to buy wheat free bread but I have not found one that is satisfactory. They are all made from commonly eaten grains, which must be avoided. In addition, they may contain yeast or lactose or sugars or unspecified vegetable oils. So I can only recommend that you stay with the uncommon grain mixtures, as described.

If after a couple of weeks your skin is not improving, it is likely to be one of the grains causing the trouble. Cut them all out and stick to the meat and vegetables only for four weeks.

◇◇◇

Providing that you are not allergic to one or more of these foods, your skin should begin to clear after about five to seven days. But food allergy and intolerance is the most bizarre and capricious thing, varying from one person to another just as our features and personalities vary.

Even innocuous things like cabbage and carrot can provoke a nasty reaction in some people. So be alert. Keep a diary of everything you have eaten, and note the reaction.

If you have an accident in the kitchen, causing contamination of your food, or if you knowingly have something you shouldn't (a chocolate, a glass of sherry, a slice of bread) it will set you back five days. If you become ill in another way, by catching a cold or 'flu, it will set you back also. But don't take any patent medicines because they will set you back far more than the infection.

If your skin begins to clear, rejoice, and stay strictly on the diet for at least four weeks before you start re-introducing foods.

However, if after a week or two there is no improvement, or very little, the reason is probably to be found in one or more of the 30 foods that you are eating. In which case I suggest that you try the three-foods diet for approximately a week.

THREE FOODS DIET

This is a much more rigid diet and requires a great deal of will-power to undertake. It will depend upon the severity of your eczema and whether or not you are desperate enough to want to try it.

If you are food allergic this diet will be effective.

Select *one only* from the following groups:

1.   Fresh lamb, free range pork or turkey, venison or any rare meat.

You *must* eat the fat from the meat

2.   Organically grown carrot, swede, turnip or sweet potato (not Irish potato).

3.   Organically grown cabbage, brussel sprouts, kale, brussel tops, cauliflower or broccoli. No spinach.

4.   Bottled water only for drinking and cooking. Coarse sea salt. No gravy thickeners. No vegetable oils.

Make a meat stock from marrow bones and any bones from the meat you eat. Boil for many hours. The broth can be a soup or just drunk from a cup – if you can only drink water, it makes a nice change. If you go out, you can take a hot flask to drink whilst others are having coffee. A generation ago, the 'stock pot' was a common sight on every kitchen range. You will need the nutrients from the marrow fat whilst you are on the three-food diet.

If you need a sweet drink, add a little glycerine to your water.

If you are meat allergic, you will not be able to tolerate this diet, in which case I would recommend that you should look into the possibility of desensitisation.

You will need to stay on this diet for five to seven days before you see any improvement in your skin. It may seem a bit dull, but in fact it is a perfectly adequate diet containing sufficient protein, fats, carbohydrate and roughage to keep you going for a long time.

It is unfashionable these days to say you need to eat the meat fat, but you will not be taking any fat from dairy produce, eggs, fish, nuts, beans, grains or vegetable oils and fatty acids are essential to the body.

After five to seven days on this three-foods diet your skin should be feeling a little easier. Do not expect a dramatic improvement, especially if the eczema has been very severe or of many years duration. I only said "a little easier". If the skin does not feel easier after five to seven days, one of the following will be the reason:

1. By an unlucky chance you have selected one of the foods to which you are intolerant. If you change to another combination you might have better luck. If not, and if you are determined to succeed and have phenomenal will-power (I never said it was easy, did I?), you can try a third combination, but each time you will have to start the five days all over again.

2. If your skin is really no better after three tries, you can be sure that you are not food allergic, *unless:*

- You have been consuming or sucking something in addition to the three foods.

- Contamination has occurred in the kitchen.

- You have reduced your steroid cream too quickly causing your skin to deteriorate from a withdrawal effect.

- If you did not purchase organically grown meat and vegetables it could be that you are chemically allergic.

- Perhaps you are taking some medicine or drug to which you are allergic.

- It is possible that you are severely allergic to inhaled or contact irritants as well as food. (I am assuming you have no animals. No-one with eczema can risk animals in the home.) You *must* pay attention to your living environment as well as foods.

- You could be sickening for something such as cold or 'flu. Anything, even a bad tooth, can make the skin worse.

- Some worry, tension or unhappiness has caused your skin to flare up.

- You have developed an infection in the skin. This can happen at any time with severe eczema.

- You have a fungal infestation of the skin or gut, which should be investigated.

No improvement at all, if none of the above possibilities has supervened, could mean that you are not food allergic and you should abandon the idea of dieting.

However, eczema is most certainly of allergic origin and it would be worthwhile looking closely into the possibility of environmental allergies, contact or inhaled, or chemical allergy, all of which are outside the scope of this book. It would be worth also looking into desensitisation.

Assuming your skin is beginning to look and feel better after about a week of the three-foods diet, you must expand your intake. These foods only are far too limited to continue for longer. You could, in fact probably would, begin to develop a new allergy to one of these three things.

Start again on the 30 food diet and see if, with the help of your diary, you can trace what had been causing the trouble before. If you are alert you will probably be able to do so. Indicative of food allergy is redness or tingling around the mouth immediately after, or whilst, eating, so watch out for this. Equally, a feeling of a bloated stomach, being over-full, unrelated to the quantity eaten, implies food allergy. Also a raised pulse immediately after eating suggests food allergy. Mouth ulcers suggest food allergy also.

Be extra careful about inhaled or contact allergens in your environment. The inhalation of perfume or the fumes from modern cleaning products could cause your skin to flare up. Contact with mould or animals or dust could have the same effect. Anything like this would confuse your assessment of the benefits of the elimination diet.

As you improve you will be able to tolerate more. It is possible that the three-foods diet for a week broke the cycle of foods damaging your skin and you can tolerate most of the 30 foods now. There is no certainty or predictability about these things. Perhaps you would prefer to start with the three-foods diet if your skin is very bad and not test the 30 foods first. It is entirely up to you how you prefer to go about things.

Continue the 30 foods diet for at least four weeks. Eczema is slow to respond, especially if it has been severe for years and the continuous use of steroid creams has damaged the skin, causing it to become thinner.

No-one would claim that this limited list of foods makes for an exciting diet. But don't let your mind dwell on that. Think positively always. Thank God for every improvement and think ahead to greater improvements. Enjoy what you *can* eat. Don't crave what you cannot have – that path only leads to frustration and dissatisfaction. Far more boring than the diet, I assure you, are the countless well-meaning folk who say, "But don't you find such a diet terribly boring?" As though it had never occurred to you!

Imagine that you have been cast away on a desert island. You crawl out of the sea half-dead with starvation. On that island you are overjoyed to find, say 15-20 varied and nutritious foodstuffs. Would you complain? Not at all, you would regard yourself as very fortunate. Perhaps the feeling of deprivation is only because our civilisation has artificially made available for us, through production, transportation, preservation, etc., things that would not naturally be available in our immediate environment. A couple of centuries ago our forefathers would certainly have regarded 30 different foods as a wide and varied diet.

The diet may not be a gastronomic delight, but it is effective. Your skin will gradually begin to clear. If you have had a few accidents or set-backs for any reason it will take proportionately longer – five days in each case. If your skin is very bad, or the eczema has been very long-standing, you may need six to eight weeks on the diet, but be of good cheer. It will overcome the eczema in the long run.

A word of warning. If you start this diet and get fed up with it after a couple of weeks, and go straight back onto your previous diet, you could make your skin much worse than it had been previously and, in addition, you could feel very ill after eating: dizzy, faint, headache, nausea, there are many possible symptoms.

This will be because the short period of abstinence has unmasked a hidden food allergy. You will have **increased sensitivity to allergenic substances** and the body will not be able to cope.

If you do abandon the diet, it would be much wiser to start your normal diet gradually, as on the re-introduction basis. However, if you suspect that you will not have the staying power to complete the four weeks on an admittedly very strict diet, it would be much better not to attempt it in the first place.

⌘

Chapter 10

WHY NOT?

Helping to unravel the mystery of why certain foods are harmful to some people.

In this chapter I want to consider foods in groups and the reasons why, as far as is known, certain things are a source of allergy to so many people with eczema. Merely to state that certain foods are best, leaves so many queries in people's minds. You need to know why.

It must be remembered though that there is no such thing as a safe food for all eczema sufferers, just as there is no food which causes trouble in all sufferers. Anyone can be allergic to anything. The following observations are just intended as general guidance.

Milk and eggs
If meats are the most widely tolerated foods, why is it that milk and eggs are among the most highly allergenic foods? After all they are animal foods also.

The answer may be that they are not animal flesh. Milk in the animal world is a baby food. The adult animal does not live on it. Human beings are the only species in the animal world that continue to drink milk into adult life, and this the milk of another species of animal.

A large proportion of the population is milk-allergic, possibly due to a relative deficiency of the enzyme lactase. The allergy is well masked because we drink so much milk every day. But none the less, the allergy remains. It causes a wide variety of illness, including eczema.

If milk is so widely allergic and known to be so why is it not always eliminated from the diet? It seems so simple.

In fact, it is not simple at all. It is extremely complicated. Thousands of people have tried what they imagine to be a milk-free diet with no benefit. They and their doctors assume that milk plays no part in the eczema and abandon the trial. This is not the case. Milk plays a large part, but the trial was not adequately or accurately carried out.

Two errors are common:

1. Milk allergy is not the *only* allergy. The others must be found and eliminated at the same time.

2. The supposed milk elimination was not an elimination diet at all but a *reduced* milk diet. This will do no good at all.

To imagine that milk reduction will control your eczema is just self-deception. Every trace of milk, and anything containing milk, must be excluded. This includes:

Cheese, butter, margarine, yoghurt, ice-cream, creams, crème fraîche, custard, chocolate

and all manufactured foods containing:

Lactase, lactic acid, lactalbumin, casein, whey, milk solids, milk protein, dried skimmed milk.

Goat and sheep's milk should not be used as a substitute as there may be a cross-reaction to cow's milk that some people cannot tolerate. Certain proteins are common to all milks.

Eggs
Eggs are not just baby food, they are foetal food upon which the unborn chick is nourished. A large number of people cannot tolerate them. In fact eggs quite commonly produce an immediate allergenic reaction in some people which can be very severe.

The fact that milk and eggs are eaten daily in one form or another by most people with no apparent ill effect is neither here nor there. If you have atopic eczema or asthma or any other allergy-related disease the possibility of a masked food allergy to your consumption of milk or eggs is very high indeed. Egg is present in a wide variety of manufactured foods, for example all cakes contain egg.

Many people are also allergic to chicken and this may be due to a cross-reaction with eggs.

Wheat, corn and grains
Wheat allergy is just as commonly a cause of eczema as dairy produce. In fact, dairy produce and grain allergies are probably the two most common causes of eczema and *both* are usually found in the same patient.

Wheat allergy is a misnomer leading one to think that wheat alone causes the trouble. This is not the case. All cereal grains are very allergenic, including:

> wheat, maize (corn) – the most troublesome
> barley, rye oats, sugar cane
> millet, rice – cause problems less commonly

Grains derive from grasses. If you have hay fever caused by grass, you are likely to have a food allergy to grains.

To eliminate every trace of cereal grain from our Western diet is just as difficult as eliminating dairy produce. What commercially prepared food can you buy these days that does not contain one of the grains, milk, eggs or sugar? Very little. That is why you must eat no packaged foods in the elimination phase of the diet.

Even if grain is not an obvious part of the food (as bread or biscuits) you will find it is a hidden ingredient in almost every food or soft drink available for purchase, often as maize (corn) derived sugar. Any ingredient which ends .....ose (eg. glucose, dextrose, lactose, fructose) can be assumed to be maize (corn) derived.

Corn allergy is just as serious and just as common as wheat allergy. Every trace of both must be eliminated from the diet.

Gluten

It must be remembered that wheat allergy is not the same as gluten allergy, which is the cause of coeliac disease. Gluten is the protein of the wheatgerm, which can be isolated and removed. You can buy gluten-free bread but eczema sufferers will not be able to take it because it remains wheat bread from which only the gluten has been removed.

Sugars

Sugars have always been used in man's diet, but in small quantities restricted by availability and seasons. However, cane sugar is new, having been introduced only in the last few hundred years. It is highly concentrated sugar and the supply is virtually unlimited. It is highly addictive and over indulgence has brought about many diseases.

All sugars including honey, jams, preserves, pickles, fruit juices, sweets, chocolates, must be eliminated. Carbohydrates, which the body breaks down into sugars, must be restricted.

Yeast

Yeast also contributes to Candidiasis.

Yeast can be very allergenic to some people. It is found naturally in a wide range of foods and is also used in the manufacture of many other foods.

Here are some of the sources:

- ☐ All breads, also buns and doughnuts
- ☐ Anything labelled "hydrolysed vegetable protein"
- ☐ Gravy powders and cubes, Oxo, Bovril, Marmite, etc.
- ☐ Beer, wine, cider and spirits
- ☐ All vinegars; all fermented food and drinks.

Naturally occurring yeast is found in:

- ☐   Cheese, especially soft creamy cheese
- ☐   Yoghurt and sour cream
- ☐   Synthetic creams
- ☐   Soy sauce
- ☐   Malt and anything labelled "malt extract"
- ☐   Commercial fruit juices
- ☐   Dried fruits
- ☐   Over-ripe fruits
- ☐   Unpeeled fruit.

In addition any left-over food kept for a day or two will develop yeast naturally, even if kept in a fridge.

If it is suspected that Candidiasis is in part the cause of your eczema, you will have to eliminate all yeast and sugars from your diet as well as having anti-fungal treatment as prescribed by your doctor. An anti-fungal diet and treatment can have a dramatic effect upon a wide range of illnesses. You may have to stay on a very low sugar diet for the rest of your life.

Other fungal foods
Moulds and fungus are well known to be an irritant to eczema through contact or inhalation. Mushrooms and puffballs are very allergenic if eaten.

Quorn and tofu and mycoprotein, which are eaten a lot by vegetarians as a protein supplement, are high in natural fungi. Truffles come into this category, but I have never met anyone who regularly eats truffles.

Sea Foods
In some people, sea foods, especially molluscs, shell fish and crustaceans, produce anaphylaxis (immediate food allergy reaction) which can be very severe indeed. Most people who suffer from this condition are aware of it. These people are usually intolerant of fish

also. This is an example of where allergy and intolerance can exist in the same person. Hidden or masked reactions to fish will need to be uncovered by the elimination diet.

It is advisable to avoid sea foods during the elimination phase and then re-introduce fish (preferably a cartilaginous fish).

If you can tolerate fish you will be able to take marine oils such as cod-liver oil or halibut-liver oil. These contain vitamins A and D, and also essential fatty acids (unsaturated) which are valuable to people who have the dry skin of eczema.

If you cannot tolerate fish you will not be able to take marine oils.

Fruit and vegetables containing pips, seeds or stones
"It seems to be the pippy things that cause the trouble." I have heard several doctors make this remark.

They are quite right – pippy things are highly allergenic to some people and there seems to be a particular link between these foods and eczema. Eliminate them from the diet and the patient's skin frequently improves.

Many doctors tell patients to eliminate some fruits, particularly citrus fruits and berry fruits. But total elimination of all fruits and vegetables containing pips, seeds or stones would be more effective.

If you have ever had hay fever caused by tree pollens you are likely to be fruit allergic.

The most widespread allergies in fruits are:

citrus fruits – oranges, tangerines, mandarins, clementines, grapefruit, lemons, limes.

berry fruits – strawberries, raspberries, loganberries, blackberries, gooseberries, cranberries, mulberries and new hybrid varieties; blackcurrants, red currants, white currants, rosehips.

81

These fruits are the most commonly associated with allergies.

Other fruits can be troublesome to some people, particularly those who have a latex allergy, because nearly all tree fruits and also tree nuts are related to the rubber tree family. (See Plant Families pp88-89.)

dried fruits: currants, raisins, sultanas, dates, figs, prunes, apricots, pears, apples.

All dried fruits are far more allergenic than fresh fruits. The drying process, unless the packet specifically states that the fruit (or vegetable) has been "sun dried", will have been dried by some chemical process, usually sulphur dioxide or a related chemical and probably other chemicals sprayed on or added to the substance before it reaches the packet stage.

Incidentally, sulphur dioxide affects the airways of some susceptible people and can provoke an asthma attack. It is not known what it will do to eczema but as there is so close a link it is not impossible that sulphur dioxide may have some effect upon the skin.

Dried fruits are high in salicylates, sugars and yeast.

Vegetables containing pips or seeds
Marrows, courgettes, cucumbers, gherkins, peppers, aubergines, chillies, tomatoes, pumpkin, squash, eggplant and many herbs and spices, particularly oriental spices; Peas and beans and this includes all dried beans and peas, pulses or lentils. All pulses are high in lectins. In some people these are incompatible with the natural lectins of the body cells.

They must all be eliminated in the first phase of the diet.

Soya Beans
These deserve special mention. They are known to be widely allergenic. Babies with milk allergy often have soy allergy also.

You must eliminate all traces of soy which is used as a flavouring in many products. It is also widely used by the pharmaceutical industry as a starch base for tablets and it is used in the manufacture of many vitamins.

Any commercially prepared food which states it contains "vegetable starches" will usually mean a soy content.

Nuts

Almost everyone knows that peanuts can be dangerously allergenic to some people, causing anaphylactic shock and even death.

If you suspect such an allergy in yourself do not touch them and in fact avoid all nuts because there is a cross-reaction link between all the nut families.

Onion family

Onions can be a problem for some people, which is not surprising when you consider what simply peeling an onion will do to the eyes of almost everyone. Of the family garlic and leek seem to be the best tolerated but it is wisest to leave them all out of the diet, in the initial stages.

If you have an overgrowth of candida, fresh garlic is highly beneficial because it inhibits the growth of yeast organisms.

Potatoes

Potatoes are highly allergenic for some people. They are relatively new to the Western diet, having been introduced from South America only about 250 years ago. Perhaps it is because we eat them so much – daily in most cases – that many people cannot tolerate them. They, and the whole potato family, must be eliminated at first, and tomatoes and peppers. Potato crisps are very allergenic.

Vegetable Oils

Specialists in food allergy advise olive or sunflower oil, but not too much.

In the initial elimination diet you should avoid maize (corn) oil or groundnut oil. Anything that is labelled "a blend of vegetable oils" should be avoided in order to make sure that any corn allergy is fully unmasked for diagnostic purposes.

Salicylates

Salicylate is found in the bark of the willow tree and from it aspirin has been developed. It is a very effective drug but is allergenic to some people with eczema. If you want to test this, take a couple of aspirins. If you turn bright red and start itching all over within 20 minutes, you will see what I mean.

Salicylate is present in just about every patent medicine for coughs, colds, 'flu, headaches, sore throats, etc., that you can buy. You will not be able to take any of these and beware of giving them to children with eczema.

Salicylates in foods

Many plant foods contain minute quantities of salicylate. There seems to be a special connection with fruits, especially the berry and dried fruits.

There also seems to be a connection with hot spicy foods. Apparently a vegetable curry will contain about 500-600 times more salicylate than the same vegetables cooked but not curried, so beware of the Indian addiction.

Stimulant drinks

Tea, coffee, coffee substitutes, soft drinks and fizzy fruit drinks and so-called natural fruit juices, chocolate, herb teas, fruit teas – in fact everything that flavours water – must be eliminated at first. The main reason is because they have all been manufactured and you cannot know what has gone into the manufacturing process.

Alcohol

All alcoholic drinks and all bottled drinks must be eliminated initially. This is because of the yeast, sugar, grain and fruit content. There are also a great many unnamed additives in alcoholic drinks.

You should also exclude home-made wines and beers because of the yeast and sugar in them.

The only safe thing to drink, I have found, is water!

Cheer up! It won't be for long. Once your skin clears and you start re-introducing foods you can experiment with drinks also, and you may be pleasantly surprised.

⌘

Chapter 11

GUIDE TO THE RE-INTRODUCTION OF FOODS

Understanding how to re-introduce foods into the diet for a successful outcome and the dangers of indiscriminate re-introduction.
Food families and cross-reactions.

When your skin is substantially improved; when you look and feel better, and the itch is subsiding; above all when you are sleeping better – then is the time to start re-introduction.

Two things need to be considered:

1. **The longer you stay on the diet and the greater the mprovement in consequence, the easier it will be to re-introduce foods.**

On the other hand:

2. **You will need more variety in your diet or you will develop new allergies.**

It can be hard to decide which is the most important. I incline to the opinion that if your skin is feeling comfortable, leave well alone and do not provoke a flare up by re-introducing too soon.

Before starting to re-introduce foods, have available the following mixture:
Soda bicarbonate: two teaspoons dissolved in a little water
Potassium bicarbonate: one teaspoon dissolved in a little water.

If, on trial, you eat something to which you have a bad reaction, take the above mixture four-hourly and a lot of water to drink until symptoms disappear. It will cut down the symptoms and general nasty effects from three days to 24 hours. (Potassium bicarbonate is obtainable from S.M. Loveridge, Southbrook Road, Southampton, SO15 1BH, telephone 023 8022 8411. It is not readily available in chemist's shops but they supply to individual customers.)

You need to re-introduce first the things to which you are *least* likely to be allergic. Do not try at an early stage anything to which there has been a positive reaction to any test you may have had. Do not test anything which is known to give you an allergic reaction, such as swelling of the mouth, tongue or throat; redness or tingling around the lips; or asthma.

Remember that your favourite foods and things you eat most frequently are going to be your most likely allergens, so leave them till last.

Do not take any commercially prepared foods or drinks during re-introduction. They will certainly contain chemical additives.

After elimination there will be an increased sensitivity in your body. If you eat something that provokes an allergic response, in addition to a skin flare up it would make you feel ill in other unexpected ways, for example, headache, shivering, palpitations, lethargy, aching limbs, sluggish or confused thinking. There are literally dozens of different reactions, and everyone responds differently. Do not think that you have caught a virus infection or something like that. It could be the food that is causing the trouble and you must stop eating it at once. Take the bicarbonate mixture four-hourly (this helps restore the pH balance in your body) and rest, if possible, until the unpleasant effects pass.

It takes at least four days for the bowel to be emptied of food residue, therefore you can take only one new food every fifth day. Reaction could occur within half an hour of eating, or it might not occur for two or three days. You cannot allow, therefore, two foods to overlap during this four day period. You would not know which had caused the trouble, and both would have to be tested again.

Patience is needed. Do not try to hurry. Eczema is a serious disease and if you are curing it by attacking the cause, do not jeopardise the result by trying to hurry back to a "normal diet".

Whilst you are re-introducing it is helpful to have available a list of food families. If you are allergic to one or two foods in a family it is likely that they will all, in that family, cause a similar reaction.

PLANT FAMILIES

Fungi or Moulds: Baker's yeast (hence breads, doughs, etc.), brewer's yeast (hence alcoholic beverages), mushrooms, truffle, chanterelle, cheese, vinegar (hence pickles and sauces.)

Grasses: Wheat, corn, barley, oats, millet, cane sugar, bamboo shoots, rice, rye, maize (note that buckwheat is not a member of the grass family).

Lily: Onion, asparagus, chives leek, garlic, sarsaparilla, shallot.

Mustard: Broccoli, cabbage, cauliflower, Brussel sprouts, horse radish, kohlrabi, radish, swede, turnip, watercress, mustard and cress, spring greens, kale, Chinese leaves.

Rose: Apple, pear, quince, almond, apricot, cherry, peach, plum, sloe blackberry, loganberry, raspberry, strawberry.

Pulses or Legumes: Pea, chick pea, soy bean, lentils, liquorice, peanut, kidney bean, string bean, haricot bean, mung bean, alfalfa, all dried beans, carob.

Citrus: Oranges, lemon, grapefruit, tangerine, clementine, ugli, satsuma, lime.

Cashew: Cashew nut, mango, pistachio.

Grape: Wine, champagne, brandy, sherry, raisin, currant, sultana, cream of tartar.

Rhubarb: Buckwheat.

Parsley: Carrot, parsley, dill, celery, fennel, parsnip, aniseed.

Nightshade: Potato, tomato, tobacco, aubergine, pepper (chilli, paprika).

Gourd: Honeydew melon, watermelon, cucumber, squashes, cantaloupe, gherkin, courgette, pumpkin.

Composite: Lettuce, chicory, sunflower, safflower, burdock, dandelion, camomile, artichoke, pyrethrum.

Mint: Mint, basil, marjoram, oregano, sage, rosemary, thyme.

Palm: Coconut, date, sago

Havea Brasiliensis: (latex rubber plant) – papaya, fig, mango, avocado , banana, chestnut, passion fruit, kiwi, melon, pineapple, peach, apricot, grape, almond.

Walnut: Walnut, pecan. (All nuts cross-react).

Goosefoot: Spinach, chard, sugar beet, beetroot.

Sterculia: Chocolate (cacao bean), cocoa, cola nut.

The following have no commonly eaten relatives: juniper, yam, vanilla, black pepper, hazelnut, maple, lychee, tea, coffee, brazil nut, ginseng, olive, sweet potato, sesame (also as tahini).

ANIMAL FAMILIES

Bovines: Cattle (beef), milk and dairy products, mutton, lamb, goat.

Poultry: Chicken, eggs, pheasant, quail (not turkey).

Duck: Duck, goose

Swine: Pork, bacon, lard (dripping), ham, sausage, pork scratchings.

Flatfish: Dab, flounder, halibut, turbot, sole, plaice.

Salmon: Salmon, trout.

Mackerel: Tuna, bonito, tunny, mackerel, skipjack.

Codfish: Haddock, cod, ling (saith), coley, hake.

Cartilaginous: Skate, ray, monkfish, dogfish (roc), shark.

Herring: Pilchard, sardine, herring, rollmop.

Molluscs: Snail, abalone, squid, clam, mussel, oyster, scallop, all shellfish.

Crustacea: Lobster, prawn, shrimp, crab, crayfish.

➤ The following commonly eaten animals and fish have no commonly eaten relatives: anchovy, sturgeon (caviar), whitefish, turkey, rabbit, deer (venison).

PLAN YOUR OWN PROGRAMME
Re-introduction can be planned to suit yourself. It does not have to follow any established order, but try to avoid re-introducing foods of the same family too close together. It is best to leave about 10 to 14 days between eating two closely related foods.

I give below a few comments which might prove helpful, but which are not intended as a chronological guide for re-introduction.

Water
You have been drinking only bottled spring water for some weeks. This is expensive and, unless you positively prefer it and intend to continue, you will want to phase it out and replace it with tap water. You will have to re-introduce water on a five-day trial basis, like any other food, to test whether or not tap water affects you adversely. I suggest you do it gradually, say half and half at first. Total change

from spring water to tap water might be a shock to the body. People who are chemical-allergic will react more sharply than those who are not.

PLANT FOODS

Grains

If you have been taking the uncommon grains mixture, as advised earlier, with no trouble you can try the commonly eaten ones. I suggest you try rice or oats or barley first. If these cause no trouble, try the others (wheat, maize, rye) with caution and the bicarbonate mixture ready to hand!

It is strange, but white bread seems better tolerated than brown wholemeal bread. This is possibly because the wheat germ has been removed. Highly refined French bread is best tolerated of all. White rice is better tolerated than brown rice for the same reason. Pasta made from durum wheat is generally better tolerated than pasta made from anything else.

On the other hand, white flour contains a huge number of chemical additives (over 50). Brown flour still contains additives, but fewer (about 20). People who are chemically sensitive will be better with wholemeal bread. French bread may be best tolerated because the French government has banned use of all additives in their flour. So French bread contains neither wheat germ nor additives.

Remember that bread contains yeast and you may have a candida overgrowth, so the yeast in the bread would cause trouble for you even if the wheat does not. Re-introduction of foods is not a straightforward affair. There are many pitfalls.

If you have been eating just meat and vegetables, with no added carbohydrates, I suggest you start grain re-introduction by taking the uncommon grains mixture.

However, if you have a bad reaction it would indicate that you are allergic to all grains and seeds and I doubt if you would be able to take *any* commonly eaten grains or seeds at all. In which case, try sago and tapioca separately. Neither are true grains. Sago is made from the pith underneath the bark of the palm tree; tapioca is made from the cassava root. If you are severely grain allergic, I recommend desensitisation.

Yeast
It is surprising how many commercially prepared foods contain yeast. The candida spores feed on yeast, and as candida is so closely linked to allergies I advise leaving out yeast and sugars indefinitely.

Vegetables
A few vegetables remained outside your diet. Try a little potato, but do not eat the skin. Do not test the close relatives tomato, pepper or aubergine within the same week.

Of the onion family, try garlic or leek first. I do not advise raw spring onions or chives at all. Try a little cooked onion later. If you can chew raw garlic, and the family will put up with you, do so. It helps overcome a fungal infestation.

Pippy vegetables
Fresh marrow and courgettes are fairly safe; fresh peas and beans also. More intolerance seems to be connected with dried peas and dried beans and pulses. It may be the drying process that alters the molecular structure or the drying has been chemical.

Soya beans are widely know to be allergenic. Try a little soya milk to see what happens. If you are allergic to soya there is a strong chance that you will react to the other pulses.

Chickpeas seem best tolerated in this family of dried legumes.

Salad vegetables
These are eaten raw. Test them separately, and be wary of raw foods.

Herbs

Most herbs and spices are known to be allergenic for some people. Try them with caution. Commercially prepared herbs and herb teas contain a lot of additives.

Mushrooms

As these are a fungus, try with caution.

Fruits

Most fruits are eaten raw. Try them and if you get a reaction try cooking them. Any fruit can be cooked, even bananas or peaches. Cooking destroys certain properties in fruit that many people with eczema cannot tolerate. Rhubarb is usually well-tolerated.

Dried Fruits

These are more likely to provoke a reaction than fresh fruits. This may be due to the drying process or because the salicylate content is much higher in dried fruits than in the fresh fruit.

Sugars

You will probably have to be very sparing with sugars and yeast for the rest of your life. This is because of the candida association with allergies.

Cane sugar, which is used in just about everything these days, is best avoided altogether along with syrup and treacle. Your safest options are the uncommon sugars such as maple syrup or palm sugar, but never too much.

If you can eat fruit try fructose, but not if it has been made from maize (corn).

Honey is highly allergenic for some people and this fact has been known for centuries.

Do not take artificial sweeteners like Sweetex and Candarel. They are chemically prepared and you do not know what you will be ingesting. If you must have something sweet take glycerine. This will do you no harm at all because it is made up of only three carbon molecules.

Nuts
Many people know that they cannot tolerate nuts, especially peanuts. If you know of such an allergy, keep away from them. If you never had a bad reaction try walnuts first. If you are latex allergic, do not try nuts.

Spicy foods
Curries and all hot spicy foods are best avoided in the re-introduction phase.

ANIMAL FOODS

Fish
White fish can be tricky for people with eczema. Test by trying a little of several different types of fish at first. This is better than a large amount of one fish. A kedgeree can be made by taking two or three ounces each of five or six different types of fish.

Cartilaginous fish are better tolerated than bony fish, generally.

Avoid smoked or dried fish because of the colouring added.

Some people have a known allergy to shell fish, molluscs or the crab family. If you know of this do not try them, otherwise try with caution. Allergy to shellfish will suggest intolerance of other fish, so be careful.

Eggs and chicken
Try the yolk of a hard-boiled egg first. If no reaction, try the white. If you can take eggs you will be lucky because they are strongly implicated in the cause of eczema.

Chicken is associated with eggs in food allergy, related to eczema. Try it with caution. But do not eat battery-reared chicken. These birds are full of drugs and toxic chemicals.

Beef
This is the only meat I had left out of the elimination phase because of its association with milk. Unless you have some other reason for not eating beef try it, freshly cooked and in moderation. Do not try beef burgers or sausages etc. because of the additives and wheat content.

Offal
Heart is recommended because it is a muscle.

Kidneys and liver are not recommended, however, I have encountered no trouble by eating them.

Ham and bacon
These can be tried, probably with success if you can eat pork. However, do not try them at all if you cannot eat pork.

Beware of ham that is coated in yellow breadcrumbs – the crumbs could make you ill.

Most bacon has a production stamp on the rind, usually in red. You must cut this out because it is an unknown dye.

Dairy produce
Milk should be tried with caution. Try goat or sheep milk first to assess the reaction. If your skin reacts badly there is no point in trying cow's milk at all.

Carnation Milk is reputed to be tolerated by people with milk allergy because it is boiled to such a high temperature that the proteins are destroyed. Try a little diluted.

Hydrolysed Baby Milk is obtainable; try a little if you like.

Try milk substitutes:
Soya milk, (assuming you can take soya), coconut, almond or sago milk, rice milk or oatmeal milk are possibilities.

Butter, cheese and yoghurt
These products are better tolerated than fresh milk.

Try hard cheese, just a little at first. If you have no reaction try soft creamy cheese. However, these contain yeast which may be troublesome if you have an underlying candida infestation.

Live yoghurt can sometimes be tolerated by milk-allergic people, so try it. It would probably be best to try goat or sheep yoghurt first to assess the result. Live yoghurt is helpful in combating candida infestation of the bowel because of the lactobacillus culture in live yoghurt. However, you must have *live* yoghurt with no added flavourings or colouring.

Beverages
Tea, coffee, cocoa, herb teas, etc., alcohol, all bottled drinks, fruit drinks, etc., must all be tested as you would a new food. You cannot assume that any one of them will be safe.

Do not drink tea made from a tea-bag. This is because the paper of the bag is bleached to make it white. You will be ingesting bleach with every cup! The same applies to coffee bags or herb tea-bags. With coffee you would be safest with coffee beans, ground yourself. Instant coffee is full of additives. De-caffeinated coffee is very suspect because the process used to remove the caffeine is unnamed on the jar.

Alcohol
This seems to provoke a reaction because of the grains, fruits, sugars, yeast and the many unnamed additives. The safest are probably distilled drinks like brandy, whisky, etc.

Commercially produced foods
It is unwise to try anything pre-packed, pre-cooked, etc., until you have completed the testing of fresh foods. When you know what you can and cannot eat you will have to develop the habit of reading and interpreting all package labels. Wheat/corn, milk, eggs, sugars,

yeast and soya are present in nearly everything commercially prepared. Avoid them if you are allergic to the fresh product.

In addition nearly all packaged foods contain chemical additives of some sort. You will need to learn more about food additives. For a recommended book covering this subject contact Merton Books (see Useful Addresses).

Time span

It is best to re-introduce all foods within three months for test purposes. Prolonged avoidance of anything can lead to relative or temporary tolerance, which breaks down very quickly on repeated ingestion of the food and the allergy re-asserts itself.

Remember – you must be very careful about re-introducing foods, because of increased sensitivity after a period of abstinence.

⌘

Chapter 12
THE ROTATION DIET AND
DIETARY SUPPLEMENTS

Concerning the four-day rotation of foods

When you are well into the re-introduction of foods, you must rotate your diet. An atopic person with food allergies will develop new allergies all the time. The bio-chemistry of the body is determinedly perverse. As you eliminate one allergenic food it will find another to react against. You must guard against this happening.

Intolerance will develop to something you eat regularly and of which you eat a considerable amount. If you eat it daily a new masked allergy could develop. New allergies can develop quite quickly, in a few weeks or months only, or they may take several years. It varies widely from person to person. The only thing that can be said with certainty is that at some stage you *will* develop new allergies unless you take steps to avoid this occurrence. The tendency gets more pronounced as you get older.

It would be sad if you had cleared your eczema through eliminating foods only to have it return months or years later, caused by a new set of allergies that developed because you did not, or were not advised, to rotate the diet.

You must rotate foods on a four day basis. This allows the food to be cleared from your body before it is taken again. It is the continual presence of any one type of food in the gut that causes the strange phenomenon – the masked food allergy.

Rotation requires organisation. Firstly you must have a diary in which you note exactly what you eat at each meal. It is best if you have only three meals a day with no snacks in between as it is easier to keep track of things. It is best to eat only one or two things at a meal. If you eat about five things it will limit your diet because all of those five foods will have to be set aside for four days until you can safely eat them again. Note everything that goes into your body.

Even seemingly insignificant things like gravy thickening or oils must be noted down, and rotated. Take no commercially prepared foods, because the content is not know.

An example: if you eat carrots on Monday, you can eat them again on Saturday; cauliflower on Tuesday, then again on Sunday, and so on. Try to rotate meats, although admittedly this is more difficult because of availability of rare meats. Thickening of meat juices to make gravy must be rotated also, i.e. potato flour, sago, buckwheat, arrowroot, rice flours, will give you a four day rotation. Drinks should be rotated too, i.e. tea, coffee, chamomile, herb or root teas, each one on a four day rotation. This may seem an awful bore but it is also a challenge. It is vitally important and is the price you will have to pay for a normal skin.

Vitamins and minerals
You may need vitamin and mineral supplements, but this is a minefield and should not be taken without medical or a nutrition consultant's supervision.

Not only must you have hypoallergenic tablets, but they must all be properly used and absorbed. They must be taken in the right dosage also, as some can be toxic when consumed in excess and virtually all interact with each other in some way.

Essential fatty acids are important in eczema with the right balance between omega-3 and omega-6. Just taking evening primrose oil or cod-liver oil is not a good idea.

Minerals can be very important if you have a mineral deficiency, but you may need a blood test to ascertain this. Just consuming mineral tablets because the advertising blurb on the packet says you need them could make matters worse because excess of one mineral could result in the non-absorption of another.

I do not wish to seem negative or dismissive about vitamins and minerals. The right supplements in the right dosage can be important. But this has to be tailored to meet the needs of each individual person, and if you cannot obtain expert guidance you are better off without them.

If you are in reasonable health, apart from the eczema, you should not need supplements during the first 3-4 weeks of the diet. After re-introduction, if you find that many vital foods have to be withdrawn from your diet permanently, you will probably need supplements, but you must obtain the right professional advice.

Useful addresses are given at the end of the book.

⌘

PART IV

THE ALLERGY VOLCANO

REACTIONS

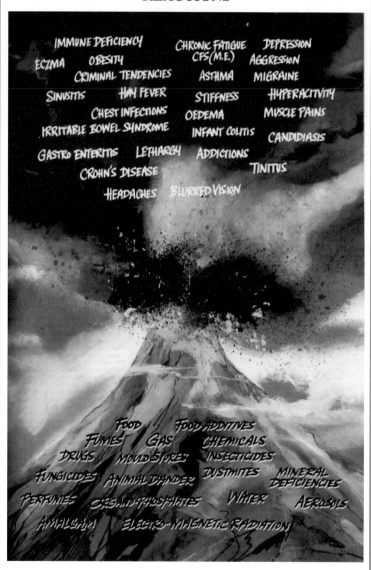

TRIGGERS

Chapter 13

THE ALLERGY VOLCANO

The allergy volcano is erupting with frightening power all over the world.

Eczema has been my main concern. But there are many other diseases of allergic origin, as the diagram graphically illustrates. Allergic conditions can affect every organ of the body:

○ The lungs and air passages

○ The digestive system

○ The articulation of joints, causing some (not all) types of arthritis

○ The skin and mucous membranes

○ The eyes, ears, nose and throat

○ The kidneys and urinary system

○ The brain – most frightening of all

Allergic conditions can render the immune system incapable of fighting infections, and some people remain ill for years following a virus infection.

Many people have multiple unidentified allergies and symptons. In such a case, the sufferer needs to see an allergy specialist, but cannot do so because the medical profession is slow to recognise the reality of allergic disease, and there are few allergy specialists in the country. Instead of getting to the root of the problem, the unfortunate patient is likely to see a chest specialist for asthma, an ENT specialist for rhinitis, a dermatologist for eczema, a rheumatologist for arthritis, a gastro-enterologist for irritable bowel syndrome, a urinologist for kidney and bladder problems, a neurologist for migraine and a psychiatrist for depression.

Each consultant will treat the symptons which are relevant to his or her specialist branch of medicine. But they will not inter-connect the whole package of symptoms. Many doctors will say that the condition of the patient is of psychosomatic origin.

Medicine is a conservative profession, for which we can all be grateful. Doctors are responsible for the health of nations and we would not want them to embrace every new product or drug unless it has been properly tested. But the trouble is that incidence of allergic diseases is galloping ahead and poor old conservative medicine is plodding along behind, not knowing quite what to make of the situation.

Relative to other branches of medicine which have been extensively researched in the last 50-100 years, allergic diseases are under-researched. Every allergy specialist I have spoken to tells me that they are seriously handicapped by lack of research. This is due to lack of money. The medical professions would welcome more money for probing into the baffling conditions caused by allergies, but they just can't get it.

Medical research is a subject that no-one knows much about. The Medical Research Council is fairly high profile, and everyone imagines it is doing its job efficiently. But in fact the MRC in Great Britain provides less that 10% of all funding for research. All the rest (and some estimate 97%) is provided by the giant international drugs companies. Whilst I have no ideological objection to private enterprise funding medical research, it must be pointed out that no drug company will pour money into something that does not produce a marketable product. A change of diet or lifestyle, reduction of chemicals in the environment, etc., will make no money for the drug companies.

The bewildering nature of allergic diseases can be seen from an article of mine which was published in *Allergy Newsletter* in December 2006, and is reproduced here by permission of the editor.

The possible effects of a viral infection on the allergic condition

A virus infection can have a devastating effect upon anyone who has an allergic condition, and I hope that my own experience can be of help to others.

Since childhood I have been allergic, having asthma, hay-fever and chronic rhinitis. About fifteen years ago I developed eczema, which covered my whole body. I discovered it was due to food allergy, and cured the eczema by a very strict elimination diet. Since then I have had EPD (Enzyme Potentiated Desensitization) which enables me to eat a normal diet, with no return of the eczema.

But the underlying allergic condition remains. Allergies never completely go away. When the body is in good health allergies can be controlled, but if anything happens to upset the balance allergies can flare up again. That is what happened to me, and it was bewildering because I became ill in a way that I had never before experienced. I did not, at first, connect it with allergy.

Shortly after New Year's Day 2006 I caught a cold. It did not seem severe enough to call it 'flu. After four or five days the cold left me, but I still felt ill, and this got worse in the days and weeks that followed. I could not understand it, because there were no asthma or bronchitis complications (probably due to cycling 1,500 miles in 2005, which strengthened my lungs). The effect was total weakness and exhaustion and perpetual tiredness, though I could not sleep. Other strange things were happening in my body: continuous headache; pains in the neck and shoulders; stiff tongue and jaw; stabbing pains in the ears; irregular heartbeat; loss of concentration; blurred vision; unsteady walk; unco-ordinated movements generally; dizziness; sleep disturbance, with alarming night sweats; kidney disturbance, similar to cystitis; muscular weakness; and worst of all a feeling of being enclosed in a bag or a sack all the time from which I could not escape.

All these unconnected symptoms do not add up to any identifiable illness known to medicine. They sound more like the ravings of a hypochondriac! But they were horribly real – sometimes I was so weak I could barely lift a kettle or walk upstairs. At one stage the pain in my neck and shoulders was so great I could not lift my arms. What was happening to me?

I was talking to my niece who is also allergic. She said "Do you think, Auntie Jenny, this could be food allergy again? Remember allergies never really go away. The viral infection you had after Christmas might have triggered it off again, and remember that allergies can change, causing new illnesses."

Why had I not thought of it? I must have been blind to the possibility. From past experience with eczema I knew just what to do – I went onto an elimination diet. For me this has to be very strict indeed: no fruit or vegetables, no cereal grains of any sort, no dairy produce or eggs, no sugar or carbohydrates, no fish. The only thing left is meat! I adopted a meat and water only diet, and within four or five days felt completely well!

Carefully I tried re-introducing foods with total failure. Anything I tried made me ill again. Fish was a disaster. I passed out on fish! My poor husband found me unconscious on the kitchen floor. However, I have a remedy given to me by a very old allergy doctor, now dead, which will reduce the worst effects of a food allergy reaction: take one teaspoonful of potassium bicarbonate* with two teaspoonfuls of sodium bicarbonate in a little water, and drink plenty; repeat four hourly until you feel better. It greatly helps with food allergy. But it does not get rid of the underlying problem, so I had to eliminate to meat and water again, and recovered again. (*See address on page 33.)

One cannot continue such an unbalanced diet indefinitely, or other problems will arise, so I saw my EPD specialist, Dr. L. E. McEwen.

He told me that the symptoms were consistent with the early stages of ME (myalgic encephalomyelitis, or chronic fatigue syndrome). He said that it was lucky for me that I had identified the source of the trouble at an early stage, because the longer it goes on the harder it is to treat. He gave me a dose of EPD vaccine that day, with instructions to continue the meat and water diet for a week, and then to re-introduce other foods slowly and in tiny quantities. About six weeks later I was back onto a full diet with no ill effects. I will have an EPD treatment every three months this year, and after that it should be all right. But I doubt it would be without EPD.

What lessons can be learned from this? Firstly, any allergic person must take a virus infection seriously, and eliminate all known allergens from the diet and environment immediately. But do not take my elimination diet as a blueprint for everyone. It is not. It is peculiar to me, and we are all different. One man's meat is another man's poison.

Secondly, expect the unexpected, because allergens shift and change all the time, and similarly allergic reactions change in a bewildering fashion.

Thirdly, consider EPD or neutralization, if possible. They are both effective. Neither of them totally cures allergies, but they greatly help.

⌘

Chapter 14

IMMUNOTHERAPY

E czema can be treated by immunotherapy, which is a form of homeopathic vaccine. There are three different types:

1 Specific Immunotherapy available on the NHS

2 Enzyme Potentiated Desensitisation (EPD)

3. Neutralization

Specific Immunotherapy dates back to 1900 and is still in use in some hospitals. It is available within the NHS.

In the 1960s two new forms of immunotherapy were developed quite independently of each other – EPD in England and Neutralization in America. Both of these methods are safe and effective and are used worldwide. Both methods must be administered by qualified doctors who are allergy specialists, trained to administer the vaccine. Most of these doctors are members of the British Society of Ecological Medicine, who can give details of practitioners. As far as I know, only the Royal London Homeopathic Hospital provides EPD treatment on the NHS. All other practitioners are private.

The chapters which follow describe these three types of immunotherapy.

Warning

Both EPD and Neutralization can only be administred by qualified doctors who specialise in allergic diseases. **Do not go to anyone who is not a qualified doctor for either of these treatments.** There are unscrupulous people around who have no medical training whatsoever, but who claim to practise immunotherapy. This is fraudulent and can be very dangerous.

⌘

Chapter 15

ENZYME POTENTIATED DESENSITISATION
Low-dose immunization
Edited by Dr Helen McEwen MBBS, MRCGP

Enzyme Potentiated Desensitisation (EPD) is very effective in the treatment of eczema. A young child will respond rapidly and usually permanently. An adult with eczema will take longer to respond. EPD is not available on the NHS.

Eczema is an allergic disease, related to asthma, hay fever, rhinitis, itchy eyes, and many other inflammatory conditions known as the 'Classical Allergic Diseases'. Allergic people have a disfunction of the immune system and a low tolerance level to allergens. To avoid all the allergens in the environment is impossible, so the only way to minimize the allergic reaction is to reduce the sensitivity to allergens. This is where EPD is effective. **It is not a drug; it is a vaccine**.

EPD is a relatively recent discovery. In the 1960s, at St Mary's Hospital Medical School in London, Dr L. E. McEwen was a member of an allergy research team. In the course of a trial to shrink nasal polyps, he observed that when **a minute dose of allergen** is combined with the **enzyme** beta-glucuronidase, the combination will **potentiate**, or induce, **desensitization**. Thus we have the tongue-twisting name!

EPD has been extensively refined during the last forty-five years, and is now used in many countries. The effect is like that of any vaccine – to build up the body's resistance over a period of time. The safety record is impressively high.

EPD is often confused with the earlier form of desensitisation called Specific Immunotherapy, but there is no connection between the two. The latter uses doses of allergen increasing with each treatment, without enzyme enhancement.

But first of all what is an 'enzyme'? The official definition is: 'a specialised protein molecule that acts as a catalyst for the biochemical reactions that occur in living cells.' In other words an enzyme is something that enables other things to happen.

Beta-glucuronidase is an enzyme present in all parts of the body, and is released into the tissues during an allergic reaction to an allergen. EPD exploits this natural phenomenon by combining a minute dose of beta-glucuronidase with a <u>minute</u> dose of allergens. The combination produces an effective desensitization technique, which has now been adapted to give an efficient treatment for most allergic diseases.

EPD has been used successfully in the treatment of:

- Asthma, eczema, hay fever, chronic rhinitis and urticaria, (known as The 'classical allergic diseases').

- Irritable bowel syndrome, ulcerative colitis and Crohn's Disease.

- Some forms of rheumatoid arthritis.

- Aching limbs, stiffness, heavy feeling, fatigue.

- Migraine, headaches, fuzzy-head feeling, memory loss and brain block.

- Childhood hyperactivity and some cases of autism.

EPD is particularly effective for the treatment of eczema. Children seem to respond after just a few doses.

I have said that minute doses are used. This is important. EPD is an extremely low-dose method of desensitizing. The actual amount of beta-glucuronidase is less than that to be found in 1cc of blood of the average person; the amount of allergen injected is less than that used for a standard skin prick test. **The dose of allergen does not increase**. Such a low dose means that a wide range of allergens can be included in each treatment. In fact about seventy different things are usually incorporated in one dose. The range can be from foods, food additives, dust, pets, tobacco, pollens, grasses, moulds, gut micro-organisms and some chemicals. The dose of each is microscopic, and alone would have no effect upon the immune system, but when combined with the enzyme the vaccine is effective.

Dealing with so many allergens at once means that the total allergy load will be treated. This is unique to EPD, and therefore the patient will not need to be tested for specific sensitivities. Most allergens cross-react with each other, and most atopic people are allergic to a wider range of allergens than they think. It follows that when EPD is used, many allergens will be cross-desensitized in groups, and unsuspected allergies will be treated.

Atopic people tend to develop new allergies all the time. This can be maddening; just when you think you have cracked one problem, another rears its ugly head. There is good evidence to suggest that, because of the wide range of allergens used, EPD protects against this problem. In other words the total allergy load has been treated, and the immune system has been strengthened overall. From personal experience I can verify this; I used to be allergic to almost everything, and now, after ten years of EPD treatment, very little affects me adversely.

Most allergens are absorbed into the body by inhalation, ingestion, or contact.

The vaccines used for EPD treatment are:

√   Inhaled and contact vaccine (The IC Mix)

√   Food, drink, and food additives vaccine (The Food Mix)

√   Special vaccines for rare allergies (The Specials Mixes)

Inhaled and Contact Mix (The IC Mix)

- ☐ House dust mites, and other mites
- ☐ Tobacco, dust, and mould spores
- ☐ Grasses
- ☐ Tree, flower, weeds, and shrub pollens
- ☐ Cat, dog and other animal fur and dander
- ☐ Respiratory tract micro-organisms.

The Food Mix contains:

- ☐ All of the above under heading IC Mix
- ☐ A wide range of common foods and drinks in the average diet
- ☐ Gut micro-organisms, including Candida
- ☐ Many of the commonly used food additives (*over 4000 food additives are currently being added to food production, and EPD cannot cover them all*).

Special EPD Mixes

In addition to the above IC Mix and Food Mix, special vaccines have been prepared to cover certain rare allergies, such as:

- ☐ Cement or building dust
- ☐ Wood dust
- ☐ Algae or rare moulds or fungi
- ☐ Mosquito and some other insect bites (but <u>not</u> wasp or bee stings)
- ☐ Some volatile chemicals.

EPD is not effective where the specific allergen cannot be identified and isolated and the last two mentioned, chemicals and latex, are examples.

Some chemicals can be identified and EPD vaccine prepared to cover them. But over five million chemicals are now recognized as being present in our environment, and they cannot all come within the ambit of EPD. Also, drug allergy cannot be covered by EPD.

Preparations before, and precautions after each dose of EPD vaccine are vitally important. If the instructions of your EPD doctor are not followed, the dose could fail, and the eczema could get worse. The principle is that **exposure to allergens must, as far as possible, be avoided for one week before and three weeks after the vaccine**. Each dose will affect the most subtle and complex part of your body chemistry – the immune system. If the body is bombarded with a high exposure to allergens just before or after the EPD dose, the immune system will react violently. Here is an example, from personal experience: I was in my second year of treatment, and had a dose of EPD in May. This is the time of year when gardeners spray their roses for fungus and black spot. A few days after the treatment, without thinking of the consequences I sprayed my roses. Later my skin, which had been perfect for about three years, broke down completely all over my body, in some parts cracking and weeping, and the itching nearly drove me mad again. My initial food allergy, which had been so much better, became worse again. It took about six months to clear up. So you can see how careful you have to be!

Food allergy contributes far more to eczema than is generally realised. You will be put onto a strict diet for at least one week before and three weeks after an EPD dose, (and possibly much longer), and this diet must be scrupulously followed. A strict anti-allergic diet can be the hardest part of all, especially for young children or teenagers who are growing and are hungry all the time. Mothers will have to be terribly careful about this and follow the doctor's instructions closely, because the wrong diet could 'blow' the whole thing, (just like my rose-spraying did for me!)

A surprisingly large number of people with eczema, including children, have a fungal disbalance of gut micro-organisms (usually called candida). Some doctors even say it is responsible for most allergies. Whether this is so or not, it is necessary for the fungal infestation to be treated before the EPD dose is given, and an anti-fungal drug will be prescribed.

Many drugs and proprietory medicines will have to be avoided before and after EPD, and a list of instructions cannot be given here. Each patient is different and will have to follow the instructions of the EPD specialist.

There are many other things that must be avoided: perfumes, hairdressing salons, air fresheners (I call them air polluters!) lavatory cleaners, and chemical perfumes/odours of all kinds, deodorants, after shave – the list could go on. Avoid dust, animals, tobacco smoke, damp buildings and mould, new paintwork and petrol fumes.

The main thing is to understand the importance of the philosophy, that **whilst your immune system is responding to the EPD vaccine, contact with known or suspected allergens must, as far as possible, be avoided.**

EPD has to be administered over a period of time. Several months must elapse between each dose. The number of doses will depend on the age of the patient and the severity of the condition. Most adults need about two years to be effectively desensitized, although some may take longer to respond. Children respond a great deal more quickly.

Before you can see an EPD specialist you will have to be referred by your own doctor. This is required procedure within the NHS, and no allergy specialist will be able to see you without a referral. If your own doctor has never heard of EPD, or refuses to refer you for any reason, ask to see another doctor in the practice. You may have to work hard at getting a referral and persistence may be necessary. All EPD consultations and treatment will have to be recorded and the details sent to your own doctor. This again, is standard procedure.

EPD is a highly individualized form of treatment in the way it is prescribed and administered. Nothing can be standardised. This means that it is only available on a 'named patient' basis (as covered by the Medicines Act.) The vaccine is only available to a registered doctor who is an allergy specialist, and who has in addition undergone a special training in the administration of EPD. The vaccine is not available to a doctor who has not been accredited, nor to a patient who does not come within the 'named patient' license of the MCA. The control of the supply of the EPD vaccine is very strict.

WARNING
Only consult a qualified doctor, accredited by the McEwen Laboratory to use EPD. I have heard of a pirate form of EPD being used by unqualified people. This is very dangerous, and could make your skin worse.

Dr L.E. McEwen, pioneer of this treatment, has retired from clinical practice, but EPD production continues and is used in Great Britain and several European countries.

There are about twenty practitioners of EPD in all parts of Great Britain. For names apply of clinics apply in writing to the McEwen Laboratory, or contact the British Society for Ecological Medicine or Action Against Allergy. *(See Useful Addresses.)*

⌘

Chapter 16`

NEUTRALIZATION
By Dr John Mansfield MRCS LRCP DRCOG

I have been treating eczema from the allergy, environmental and nutritional point of view for over 30 years.

I have seen over these years, countless eczema sufferers respond excellently following the identification and avoidance of various food allergies or intolerances. There are also, however, a lot of other fundamental causes of eczema, such as the candida yeast problem (or perhaps more accurately fungal type dysbiosis) and biological inhaled allergens such as housedust, dustmite, moulds and animal danders. Other noted causes have been chemical sensitivity and nutritional deficiencies, such as those involving zinc and essential fatty acids. Rarely, heavy metal sensitivity such as reactions to mercury from amalgams may play a role.

In patients with food sensitivity, biological inhalant sensitivity and chemical sensitivity, the use of neutralization testing and treatment can be totally critical to a successful outcome. Patients with multiple food sensitivities, especially to difficult to avoid foods, rarely do well without neutralization. Biological inhalant allergens are almost totally impossible to avoid without emigration to a hot, dry climate where dust, dustmite and moulds do not normally exist. The intradermal testing performed as part of the neutralization procedure is also the best way of identifying these problems.

Intradermal testing is also the single best method of identifying chemical sensitivities such as gas, formaldehyde and phenol.

It must be emphasised that the use of food, inhalant or chemical neutralization is equally preferable whether the patient is suffering from eczema, asthma, rhinitis, irritable bowel, rheumatoid arthritis or any other condition, which responds to these approaches.

SAFETY

With provocative neutralization therapy we observe almost total safety. There has not to my knowledge been a single fatality recorded anywhere in the world as a result of provocative neutralization therapy or testing. Currently there are only about 8 clinics using this method in the UK. There are, however, over 4,000 clinics in the US using this technique. Provocative neutralization is used as the method of choice by members of the American Academy of Environmental Medicine, the American Academy of Otolargyngolic Allergy and the Pan American Allergy Society. The combined membership of these large societies exceeds over 3,000 physicians, and all these societies run annual instructional courses for physicians interested in the technique.

At least 30 million patients, at a conservative estimate, have therefore received this form of treatment over a period of many years without any fatalities. Most of these patients were in the USA or Canada, but over one hundred thousand have also been treated in the UK and Australia.

This safety factor is not surprising when one considers that the provocation neutralization method uses doses that are frequently several thousand times weaker than those used in incremental desensitization.

The Technique of Food Neutralization

Food extracts are obtained from the usual allergy supply companies in the standard 1/10 or 1/20 prick test concentrates. These concentrates contain 50 per cent glycerine, added during the course of the extraction to stabilize the food molecules. This maintains their potency for several years. As with inhaled allergens we use benzyl alcohol in intravenous-quality normal saline to dilute these extracts (serial 1-in-5 dilutions).

In contrast to inhalant testing, with foods we normally start on the number 1 (1-in-5) or 2 (1-in-25) strengths. As the concentrate contains 50 per cent glycerine, the Number 1 strength (1-in-5) will contain 10 per cent glycerine and the Number 2 strength will contain 2 per cent glycerine. Ten per cent glycerine has a water-attracting (hygroscopic) effect and, as such, will draw fluid into the site of the wheal from the neighbouring tissue. Thus an injection of pure 10 per cent glycerine into the skin will, in most patients, produce a positive wheal reaction. This is *not* because they are sensitive to glycerine, but because of its water-attracting effect. Thus if a Number 1 food skin test is to be judged positive the wheal must grow by more than the 10 per cent glycerine control. In the case of the Number 2 level, as this contains only 2 per cent glycerine this is not enough to have this water-attracting effect.

The most common neutralizing levels for food allergens are the 2, 3 and 4 levels, which contrasts with the 4, 5, 6 and 7 levels in regard to inhalant allergies. It is this single fact, which explains, incidentally, why skin prick tests are so totally useless in diagnosing food allergies. Only about one in six food tests will be positive on the Number 4 strength, and it is the Number 4 strength which is equivalent to a skin prick test. Dr Keith Eaton discovered that prick tests in patients with known food allergies had a success rate of only 15 per cent; put another way, this means an 85 per cent failure rate. To emphasize the uselessness of skin prick testing with food allergy, one could make the point that tossing a coin will give a 50 per cent reliability and so skin prick testing is three times worse that the tossing of a coin. Countless patients, in my experience, have been told that they are not sensitive to a food on the basis of a negative prick test, even when they have been convinced from their own observations that a specific food upsets them.

The single most common neutralizing level is the Number 2 level, with the Number 3 level being the next most common. Rarely, patients may even neutralize on a Number 1 level. In these circumstances they may develop symptoms on a negative Number 2 test (indicating under-dosage), which then become relieved by giving the stronger dose, the Number 1 level. This then proves that the Number 1 is the neutralizing dose.

Diagnosis of Food Allergy by Skin Test

Most patients with food allergy are sorted out by an elimination diet; the skin testing in these patients is used only to determine their neutralizing levels to foods which have been already identified, but which need neutralization. An extension of the skin test technique is to use it for diagnosis. Clearly, if positive wheal reactions and symptoms can be obtained in the course of skin testing there is no absolute need to go through an elimination dietary procedure. Furthermore, whereas an elimination diet can take five or six weeks, during which time major social occasions may need to be avoided, a comprehensive skin testing programme can be completed in about two and a half to three days of intensive testing. A workable procedure involves scanning about 34 major foods with intradermal provocative skin tests. The reaction to all 34 foods is tested, and neutralizing doses are obtained for all those items to which there is a positive reaction. At the end of the test programme, the patient is only allowed to eat those foods tested and to take neutralizing injections to cover all those items to which a sensitivity has been found. The advantages of this approach are considerable.

√ The Test programme is completed in a few days.

√ The patient does not need to assess his or her own response.

√ There is no need to abandon drugs other than antihistamine.

√ If the patient lives a long way from the clinic the test procedure saves a whole series of long journeys at various stages of the elimination diet.

√ If multiple food sensitivities are involved, these tests will be inevitable anyway, even after the elimination diet, because it will be necessary to desensitize the patient to a large number of foods.

√ In some patients their reactions to foods are very insidious and can be picked up better by skin test.

√ In most cases the treatment programme is very successful.

The disadvantages of this treatment, as opposed to the elimination diet followed by desensitization to specifically identified food allergens, are:

- The skin test technique picks up adapted food allergies as well as non-adapted food allergies. Hence the number of foods to which someone reacts often appears more complicated than it really is, and a degree of overtreatment is almost certainly inevitable using this technique.

- Patients do not know whether they are going to see a successful outcome until after the treatment is completed, whereas after the first stage of an elimination diet most discover for themselves that, once removed from their major food allergies, they feel much better.

- Going through an elimination diet probably gives the patient a better idea than skin testing as to which food allergens cause severe reactions and which mild, and also the patient may learn to associate certain symptoms with certain foods.

- The elimination diet is an educative programme, whereas skin testing is far less so in itself. Consequently, at the end of a skin testing programme the patient must learn to use only those items which have been evaluated. This involves some education into the way in which multiple foods are made up and what they contain. For example, at the end of the testing programme it is probable that wholemeal bread will be permitted, but not white bread because the chemicals (bleaching agents, anti-staling agents, etc.) added to this have not been assessed. Thus, at the end of such a programme a patient could conceivably sabotage all the careful work that has been done up to that point by, for example, eating white bread. If the patient is sensitive to the chemicals in white bread and is not covered for them by desensitizing drops or injections, this may in itself be enough to cause symptoms to continue. This is just one example; I could give many others.

After remaining on the foods tested for a few weeks and presumably observing a huge improvement in their eczema, patients can then extend their repertoire of foods by bringing back into the diet one single food at a time and observing any response.

The fundamental principals for the treatment of inhaled allergens which cause eczema are identical, but we tend to neutralize on higher numbers, ie. 5, 6 and 7.

Administration of Neutralization
After the neutralizing levels for the major food and inhaled allergens have been determined, they are either administered to the patient by sublingual drops or by subcutaneous injections, which are usually self-administered.

Technicians use a fairly simple mathematical formula to calculate the amount of reagent each patient needs, dependent on the results of the skin testing. Sublingual drops are effective for about five hours, while subcutaneous injections will be effective for two days in most patients. The injections are normally made up in a 0.1 cc dosage; the amount of inhaled allergen in these is, of course, calculated appropriately.

Of the two methods, my preference is for the subcutaneous injections, although I do use both on my patients. Nowadays, modern insulin syringes are disposable, have a very fine in-built needle, are extremely easy to use and, most important of all, very rarely hurt the patient. Most patients who try both methods of administering their neutralizing doses prefer the injection because it is much more effective, and the fact that it is only required every two days makes it very convenient.

These desensitizing drops or injections fulfil two purposes. The first is that, within a week or so, they enable the patient to inhale aero-allergens without adverse effect. Secondly, if the desensitization has been administered for a year to one-and-a-half years, the patient becomes desensitized to these inhalants and does not need to take further desensitization treatment.

In the case of food allergies/intolerance, the injection usually enables the patient to eat such foods within one week. However, it is usually two to three years before the patient can eat incriminated foods without the injection.

Disadvantages of Neutralization Therapy

By far the biggest problem with neutralization therapy is the fact that after several weeks or months of this treatment the neutralizing levels can change. Often the specific reason for this change is inexplicable, but in many cases it appears to be a feature of the progressive desensitization that is occurring as treatment continues to be administered. What normally happens is that a patient who has experienced enormous or total relief suddenly notices that the symptoms are beginning to recur without any obvious change in the environment or diet. In these circumstances re-testing is indicated. Another possible reason for a change in neutralizing levels is the occurrence of a severe attack of flu or a similar viral illness. Whatever the reason for the change, however, re-testing is indicated. Most frequently the re-testing reveals that the neutralizing levels have become stronger. In other words, as the patient has become progressively desensitized, a stronger dose is needed to neutralize his or her symptoms. It is furthermore possible that several months later the neutralization levels will again change to an even stronger level, at which point the levels usually remain stable. Certainly, instability of neutralizing levels almost inevitably decreases with time.

The main disadvantage with changing neutralizing levels, of course, concerns the inevitable cost to the patient of re-testing and taking time off work for this to be done. If only a few inhalants are involved this is a minor problem, but it can be quite a big problem if multiple allergies are being dealt with. The ongoing cost of the neutralizing injections is comparatively small and this compares favourably with the cost of anti eczema ointments and other medications.

To find a practitioner of neutralization in the UK, contact:
British Society of Ecological Medicine
PO Box 7, Knighton, LD7 1WF. Tel: 0906 3020010.
Dr John Mansfield, The Burghwood Clinic
34 Brighton Road, Banstead, Surrey SM7 1BS. Tel: 01737 361177
or 352245.
Dr Jean Munro, The Breakspear Hospital
Wood Lane, Paradise Estate, Hemel Hempstead, Herts HP2 4DF.
Tel: 01442 261 333.
Dr David Freed, Salford Private Allergy Clinic
14 Marston Road, Salford, Greater Manchester M7 4ER. Tel: 0161
795 6225
Dr Ray Chay
11-12 Wimpole Street, London, W1G 9ST. Tel: 0207 436 2135.
Dr Stewart Morison
4 Orchard Close, Horndean, Hants PO8 9LL. Tel: 02392 593529
The Institute of Complementary Medicine
51 Bedford Place, Southampton, S015 2DT. Tel: 02380 334752.
The Dove Clinic for Integrated Medicine (Dr Julian Kenyon)
97 Harley Street, London, W1G 6AG. Tel: 0207 486 5588.

To find a practitioner in USA or Canada, contact:
American Academy of Environmental Medicine
7701 East Kellogg, Suite 625, Wichita KS 67207, USA
The Department of Integrative Medicine
Capital University, Washington, USA

To find a practitioner in Australia or New Zealand, contact:
The Australian Academy of Environmental Medicine
2/11 Howell Close, Doncaster East, Victoria 3109, Australia

To find a practitioner in Northern Europe, contact:
Fachkrankenhaus
Nordfriesland, Bredstedt, Germany

⌘

Chapter 17

SPECIFIC IMMUNOTHERAPY

by Professor Anthony Frew BChir, MB,MA,MD,FRCP

Most patients with allergic disorders would like to get rid of their allergies. When somebody is diagnosed with an allergic condition, the first thing that is generally tried is some form of allergen avoidance. Obviously for exotic foods this may be straightforward, but for common foods, or for most inhaled allergens, it can be extremely difficult for the sufferer to avoid exposure. Given a straight choice, most people would prefer not to take medication every day, but if you cannot avoid the things that cause your allergies and you have significant symptoms then regular medication with antihistamines, inhaled steroids, eye drops etc may be the only way that you can bring your symptoms under control.

In the UK, we have been reluctant to recommend desensitising injections to patients with allergic disease. This is perhaps a bit surprising as desensitisation (sometimes called Specific Immunotherapy) was invented in the UK by investigators in St Mary's Hospital, London at the end of the nineteenth century. The basic Principle is to administer increasing doses of an allergen extract to desensitise the patient and either reduce or completely abolish their response to the offending allergen. Most doctors who work in this area believe that the administration of allergen extracts helps the immune system to deviate away from the allergic response towards a more protective pattern of response. The allergic patient does not get rid of their sensitivity completely, but you can reduce the impact of the allergy and in many cases reduce the symptoms of allergic disease considerably. Put simply, this approach should help to treat the cause rather than just simply mask the problem.

Experiments with pollen
Early investigators thought that hayfever was caused by an infectious agent contained within pollen. This was why they started to look at ways of vaccinating people against pollen. Early

experiments demonstrated that even small amounts of pollen could cause quite severe allergic reactions so a dosage schedule was developed, **starting with an extremely low dose and building up gradually.** By this means the investigators were able to proceed to give a large dose of the pollen without causing an allergic response. This approach to desensitisation was enthusiastically adopted in the United States, where the principles and practice of immunotherapy were developed in hospital and office departments of allergy during the 1920s and 1930s. In the UK, desensitisation became popular in the 1950s and was widely promoted in Primary Care during the 1960s and 1970s. Towards the end of the 1970s new vaccines were developed which were more powerful than the older vaccines and caused more problems with side effects. Unfortunately, a number of patients developed severe allergic reactions to their vaccines and a few died from acute asthma. This led the Committee on the Safety of Medicines to restrict immunotherapy to specialised centres from 1986 onwards. Although desensitisation has continued in the UK since 1986, it is only available in a relatively small number of centres and has not been given full funding by the healthcare system. As a result, many patients are not aware that they can be desensitised for their problems, and indeed many GPs are not aware that the service continues to function. This sometimes leads to patients being told that there is no desensitisation in the UK any more, when in fact it remains available for appropriately selected patients.

Poor control of symptoms
Evidence that desensitisation is still needed comes from a variety of sources. A survey of 64,000 patients in Wessex found that 10% of these had been prescribed antihistamines or nasal steroids during the hayfever season. Of those receiving conventional medication for hayfever, only 35-38% reported good control of nasal symptoms such as itching, sneezing, nasal blockage and nose running. About 45% reported partial control and the remaining 10-15% reported poor control of their symptoms. Similar figures were reported for eye symptoms. Many patients with hayfever find that systemic symptoms such as irritability and tiredness are much more of a

nuisance, and among our sample only 20% of patients reported good control of these symptoms, while 28-30% reported poor control of their irritability or tiredness. Overall, this study found that about 10% of patients in our community had significant hayfever that caused them to consult their doctor. About 11% of these (i.e. just over 1% of the total population) were taking regular nasal steroids and antihistamines but only 46% reported good overall control. 15% of these had poor overall control which means that at least 600,000 people in the UK have sufficiently bad hayfever to warrant desensitisation, even by current criteria.

Careful assessment
Desensitisation is used for a number of different conditions and has been shown to be effective in allergy to wasp and bee stings, hayfever, cat allergy, asthma and even in latex allergy. Desensitisation for allergic reactions to wasp and bee stings is not a controversial issue. Indeed, desensitisation is the treatment of choice for such patients. However, the decision to treat patients for allergy to wasp and bee stings has to be based on a careful assessment of the nature of the reaction experienced, the level of risk for future exposure and the amount of antibody that the patient has directed against the venom. Protection is achieved during the first few weeks of treatment and can be maintained for at least ten years after ceasing treatment. Usually injections are given weekly for about ten weeks, followed by maintenance injections every 6-8 weeks for a total of three years. Once treated, the patient is able to go out and about and enjoy themselves without worrying about the possibility of an anaphylactic response to a sting. Alternative approaches such as giving patients injectable adrenaline (epipens) can reassure some patients but may leave people feeling vulnerable and anxious when they see a wasp or bee circling round their picnic.

Specific immunotherapy for hayfever has been shown to be effective in a number of different studies. Most recently, a large randomised study in the UK found a 40% reduction in symptoms and medication requirements when patients were treated with conventional desensitisation for just one year. It is worth stressing that this improvement was achieved in patients who had not been able to obtain control of their symptoms using conventional medication, so we can be confident in saying that this treatment offers something over and above that which is achievable with antihistamines and steroid sprays.

Allergy to cats is extremely common and presents a significant hazard to people who work in the community. There are approximately nine million cats in the UK and cats are either present in or occasional visitors to about 70% of UK homes. As well as the problem of people becoming allergic to their own cats, there are substantial social problems for people who are allergic to cats and cannot visit their relatives or carry out their duties in the community. By desensitising to cat dander it is possible to almost completely abolish the allergic response to cat exposure. Protection against cat exposure can be achieved within about six weeks but for full and lasting protection it is recommended to treat patients for at least two years, preferably three.

Where desensitisation works best
Immunotherapy works extremely well in rhinitis and conjunctivitis but also has benefits in allergic asthma. The degree of benefit in asthma is less than for nasal symptoms. We believe that this is partly because allergy is an important risk factor for asthma but it is certainly not the only thing that drives and maintains the asthmatic process. Desensitisation to grass pollen or house dust mite shows a clear benefit in terms of asthma symptom scores and allergic responses to inhaled allergens. However, the benefit for bronchial irritability is somewhat less striking. This suggests that desensitisation probably works best in patients whose asthma is primarily driven by inhalation of allergens but will be less effective in patients with multiple sensitivities or those who do not have such obvious responses to inhaled allergens.

Desensitisation has been attempted for a number of other allergens including latex and peanuts. A protocol for desensitising people to latex has been developed recently and is based on a short course of injections. The current regime has a fairly high rate of side effects and we are not yet clear how long the benefit lasts for. For these reasons, desensitisation for latex allergy remains an area of great interest but is currently the subject of research rather than something that can be recommended for routine use.

Desensitisation for foods is a very exciting area that may become possible over the next few years. Obvious targets include peanuts, tree nuts, shellfish etc. Some care is needed in this area as we need to understand whether it will be a treatment that just reduces the risk of anaphylaxis in patients who are accidentally exposed or whether we could achieve a degree of desensitisation whereby patients will be able to eat the suspect food deliberately. Nobody is yet clear whether it will be safe for people to eat the food, even if they avoid anaphylaxis. Watch this space!

Obtaining a lasting benefit
Having established the patient on maintenance treatment and achieved a degree of improvement, it is probably necessary to continue for at least two years to obtain a lasting benefit. Most centres recommend three years treatment for patients who respond but would terminate the course of treatment if there is no benefit after two years. We have good research evidence that the benefits of treatment last for at least five years after ceasing treatment. Most allergists believe that desensitisation works for at least ten years and probably longer but it is difficult to obtain good quality data. This is partly because it is difficult to follow people up for ten years or more, but also because the natural history of allergy is quite variable, with some patients showing natural resolution and others having continuing symptoms over many years. In any event, the benefits achieved within the first few years of treatment are usually appreciated by the patient and represent a valuable achievement in themselves, even if they did not last forever.

In the United States, it is customary to desensitise allergic patients with a cocktail of allergens based on the range of skin test sensitivities. This type of treatment is more difficult to assess in clinical trials than the single allergen vaccines that are generally used in Europe. Randomised trials in the United States have not shown any great advantage of the US-style immunotherapy for asthmatic children who are receiving good conventional anti-asthma drugs therapy. However, this does not mean that the immunotherapy has no benefit. Firstly, there may be some advantages in desensitising the patient and reducing the amount of anti-asthma drugs that they need to take, even if the overall benefit is limited. Secondly, it may be that this approach with multiple allergens could be refined, or indeed may be more effective in adults than it is in children.

A number of alternative routes of administration have been tried. Among these, the sublingual (under the tongue) approach is the most promising. A large number of studies have been conducted in Germany, Italy, France and most recently the UK to assess the benefits of sublingual immunotherapy. Usually these regimes involve quite large doses of grass pollen which are given either as tablets or drops under the tongue. The treatment can be given at home and so has potential advantages for the UK where it is difficult for patients to travel to find an allergy clinic where they can receive desensitising injections.

Although many people did not expect sublingual immunotherapy to be very effective, it does seem to have some benefits in terms of symptom control, especially as patients move into the second year of therapy. Local side effects are quite common (itching and irritation at the site where the tablets are given). However, generally speaking, sublingual immunotherapy seems to be very safe and does not carry the risk of anaphylactic reactions that is always there with injections.

There is now good evidence that treating children with allergic rhinitis can prevent them from developing new sensitisations. In a trial of forty four children who were only allergic to house dust mite, those who did not receive immunotherapy all went on to develop new sensitisations to cat, dog, moulds or grass pollen. In contrast, half of those who had immunotherapy showed no new sensitisations.

Studies conducted in the 1960s showed that when children with asthma were treated by immunotherapy, they were more likely to lose their asthma or to have only mild asthma by the time they reached sixteen. This data was published back in 1968 and used relatively old-fashioned extracts. A large and continuing study in Scandinavia and Germany is assessing whether the modern extracts are able to have the same effect. Five years into the study, there is a two and a half-fold reduction in the development of asthma in the children who had active treatment compared to those who had placebo. If this study continues to show the same difference and demonstrates that desensitisation for rhinitis can indeed prevent asthma as opposed to merely postponing it, then there will be a very strong case for us to start treating children with rhinitis more aggressively and desensitising them to their allergies so that we can prevent them from going on to develop asthma.

Reducing the risk

As in all areas of medicine, one of the basic principles is that any treatment you prescribe should give benefit without causing unnecessary harm. Unfortunately, desensitising injections do carry a small but definite risk of causing anaphylactic reactions and asthma.

The risk of serious adverse reactions can be reduced by selecting patients carefully, by training the staff who will administer the injections and deal with any side effects, as well as by giving anti-histamine premedication and using well standardised vaccines. All these steps are used in the UK and since the restriction to specialist centres in 1986, there have been no reported fatalities from desensitising injections. It must be acknowledged that there have been many fewer patients treated since 1986 than in the previous era. Nevertheless, it does appear that concentrating the treatment of patients with allergic disease into specialist centres has been beneficial in terms of reducing the risks of serious adverse events.

Sublingual treatment

Looking to the future, there are several areas where immunotherapy may develop. Firstly, we may see desensitisation for new allergens such as nuts, moulds, food, latex etc. The new routes, such as sub-lingual immunotherapy, may allow us to treat a wider range of patients who are not currently able to give up the time to come to the desensitisation clinics at the specialist centres. It is also possible that sublingual treatment may prove more effective for some patients and could replace conventional injection immunotherapy, but we need to see the evidence for this before making any firm decisions. Several companies are developing modified vaccines which carry a much lower risk of side effects but remain effective. These may be given as shorter courses, e.g. four weekly injections instead of three years of therapy. New vaccines using short synthetic peptides may also be effective. These are short length molecules cut out of pollen or cat protein and can influence the white blood cells that control allergic responses without having any risk of triggering anaphylaxis. Scientists are even working on DNA vaccines which might allow us to drive a completely different sort of immune response to the pollen, cat dander, mould etc. all of these developments are very exciting and should offer us new and safer ways of influencing the allergic response and helping patients with allergic disease.

In conclusion, desensitisation is a useful and effective way of controlling allergic symptoms. The benefits are real and sustained over the long term. Obviously there are costs to doing this and they have to be offset against the long term benefit rather than any immediate reduction in drug usage. Safety remains a key issue and is the spur for future development of safe standardised vaccines that we should be seeing within the next five to ten years.

This article was first published in *Allergy Newsletter No. 82, Winter 2004.* Prof. Frew has his NHS practice at the Department of Respiratory Medicine, Brighton General Hospital. He sees private patients at the Nuffield Hospital, Brighton (T: 01273 624488) and the BUPA Hospital, Southampton (T: 023 8077 5544).

⌘

USEFUL ADDRESSES

Action Against Allergy (AAA)
PO Box 278, Twickenham, Middlesex, TW1 4QQ. T: 020 8892 4949. www.actionagainstallergy.co.uk. National charity offering advice and help on all aspects of living with allergies including addresses of allergy specialists. Membership brings a thrice-yearly newsletter, an update on books and information and access to a Talkline telephone network.

Allergy UK
3 White Oak Square, London Road, Swanley, Kent BR8 7AG.. T: 01322 619898. www.allergyuk.org. There is an allergy and chemical sensitivity helpline on this number. They cannot give names of doctors over the phone.

Asthma UK
Summit House, 70 Wilson Street, London EC2A 2DB. T: 020 7786 4900. www.asthma.org.uk. Advice line with asthma nurse specialist on 08457 010203. This society offers advice and help on all aspects of living with asthma, including children's holidays. Membership is advisable.

BioCare Ltd
180 Lifford Lane, Kings Norton, Birmingham, B30 3NU. T: 0121 433 3727. www.biocare.co.uk. A science based company supplying vitamin supplements and herbal medicines, including probiotics, essential fatty acids and antioxidants. Offers information on all matters relating to nutritional medicine.

British Association for Nutritional Therapy
27 Old Gloucester Street, London, WC1N 3XX. T: 08706 061284. www.bant.org.uk. Registered for education in all aspects of nutritional medicine. Supplies contact details of qualified therapists. Specific nutritional information not available.

British Dietetic Association (BDA)
5th Floor, Charles House, 148/9 Gt Charles Street, Queensway, Birmingham, B3 3HT. T: 0121 200 8080. www.bda.uk.com. The BDA was established in 1936 to provide training for Registered Dieticians. They have a register of dieticians who have had special training in food allergy and intolerance.

British Society for Ecological Medicine (BSEM)
PO Box 7, Knighton, LD7 1WT. T: 01547 550378. www.ecomed.org.uk. Promotes the study and good practice of allergy, environmental and nutritional medicine. Supplies a list of qualified practitioners. Also offers associate membership to dentists, vets, nurses and allied professions.

British Society for Mercury-Free Dentistry
PO Box 42606, London, SW5 0XA. Help-line T: 020 8746 1177. www.mercuryfreedentistry.co.uk. Information concerning dental amalgam and its effects upon health. Also details of tests and treatments available. Provies names of dental practitioners who provide biocompatible dental materials and treatment.

British Society for Allergy & Clinical Immunology
17 Doughty Street, London WC1N 2PL. T: 020 7404 0278 www.info@bsaci.org. The professional body for allergy specialist consultants and immunologists. Supplies details of clinics where members practise.

Centre for Complementary & Integrated Medicine
56 Bedford Place, Southampton, Hampshire SO15 2DT. T: 023 8033 4752. www.complemed.co.uk. Treats private and NHS patients offering homeopathy, acupuncture, herbal and nutritional medicine. Provides information about different therapies.

Institute of Optimal Nutrition (ION)
72 Lower Mortlake Road, Richmond TW9 2JY. For information leaflet T: 020 8614 7800. www.ion.ac.uk. Education in all aspects of nutritional medicine.

Latex Allergy Support Group
PO Box 27, Filey YO14 9YH A support network for those affected by latex allergy, run by volunteers. Helpline T: 07071 225838 7pm-10pm. www.lasg.co.uk. Campaigns to raise awareness of latex health hazards. Provides a patient information sheet for latex allergics going to hospital.

McEwen Laboratories
12 Horseshoe Park, Pangbourne, Berks, RG8 7JW. T: 0118 984 1288. Dr L McEwen remains at the centre of Enzyme Potentiated Desensitization (EPD) treatment and research. His secretary will advise on a medical practitioner, licensed to carry out EPD in all areas.

Merton Books
PO Box 279, Twickenham TW1 4XQ. T: 020 8892 4949. www.mertonbooks.co.uk A mail order service offering a wide choice of books on self-management across the whole spectrum of allergic illness and many useful 'free from' recipe books for those on restricted diets. Telephone credit cards accepted and on-line shopping facility.

National Candida Society
PO Box 151, Orpington, Kent BR5 1UJ. T: 01689 813 039. www.candida-society.org. Information for people with candida overgrowth and health care professionals.

National Eczema Society (NES)
Hill House, Highgate Hill, London, N19 5NA. T: 020 7281 3553. Helpline T: 0870 2413604. www.eczema.org. Offers help and advice on living with all aspects of eczema including advice about contact and environmental allergens, clothing, bathing, moisturizing, Disability Living Allowance, Invalid Care Allowance and how to apply; children's holidays, pen friends, schooling, hobbies, etc. Members receive a quarterly magazine and regular updates.

National Society for Research into Allergy (NSRA)
PO Box 45, Hinckley, Leics, LE10 1JY. T: 01455 250715. www.all-allergy.co.uk. A registered charity founded 1980 by Eunice Rose, a knowledgeable lady, who runs a telephone helpline offering counselling, advice and information, including addresses of doctors specializing in allergies in all areas. The Society has funded several important allergy research projects. Membership is advisable. Send a large S.A.E. with any query, and a donation to cover expenses.

Royal London Homoeopathic Hospital NHS Trust
60 Great Ormond Street, London, WC1N 3HR. Tel: 020 7391 8891. Consultant Physician: Dr Saul Berkovitz, BChir,MB,MRCP,NFHom, who provides EPD treatment on the NHS and privately. (Secretary on T: 020 7391 8873.)

Soil Association
South Plaza, Marlborough Street, Bristol, BS1 3NX. T:0117 314 5000. www.soilassociation.org. Will advise on all matters of organic farming and supply addresses of organic retail suppliers in all areas of the UK.

⌘

INDEX
Main references only